HUMAN REPRODUCTIVE SYSTEM - ANATOMY, ROLES AND DISORDERS

SPERMATOGENESIS

MOLECULAR MECHANISMS, REGULATION AND BIOLOGICAL PERSPECTIVES

HUMAN REPRODUCTIVE SYSTEM - ANATOMY, ROLES AND DISORDERS

Additional books in this series can be found on Nova's website under the Series tab.

Additional e-books in this series can be found on Nova's website under the eBooks tab.

HUMAN REPRODUCTIVE SYSTEM - ANATOMY, ROLES AND DISORDERS

SPERMATOGENESIS

MOLECULAR MECHANISMS, REGULATION AND BIOLOGICAL PERSPECTIVES

GLADYS ROBINSON
EDITOR

NOVA BIOMEDICAL

New York

NOTICE TO THE READER

Library of Congress Cataloging-in-Publication Data

ISBN: 978-1-63484-715-5
Library of Congress Control Number: 2016931589

Published by Nova Science Publishers, Inc. † New York

CONTENTS

Preface		**vii**
Chapter 1	The Molecular Mechanisms Underlying Acrosome Biogenesis *Chao Liu and Wei Li*	**1**
Chapter 2	Regulatory Role of Noncoding RNAs during Spermatogenesis *Wenxian Zeng, Chuanying Pan and Wan-Sheng Liu*	**31**
Chapter 3	Testicular Immune Environment for Spermatogenesis *Tingting Deng and Daishu Han*	**71**
Index		**101**

PREFACE

Spermatogenesis is a tightly regulated cellular renovation and differentiation process. It consists of self-renewal and differentiation of spermatogonial stem cells (SSCs), spermatocytic meiosis and spermiogenesis; each of these processes is essential to the continuous, successful production of male gametes. During spermiogenesis, haploid spermatids undergo extensive cellular, molecular and morphological changes, including acrosome biogenesis, flagellum development, cytoplasmic reorganization and chromatin condensation. These changes ultimately result in mature spermatozoa with an acrosome-covered head and motile tail. In this book, Chapter One summarizes the progress that has been made in understanding the molecular mechanisms underlying acrosome biogenesis, and the authors discuss the potential directions of future investigations of this process. Chapter Two briefly addresses the basics of spermatogenesis and the synthesis of ncRNAs, and then the authors discuss the recent progress in understanding of the functions of miRNAs, endo-siRNAs, piRNAs and lncRNAs in the regulation of spermatogenesis. Chapter Three provides a review of the current literature on testicular immunoregulation and its underlying mechanisms, along with its effect on testicular functions.

Chapter 1 – The acrosome is a secretory vesicle that covers the anterior part of the sperm nucleus and is essential for sperm-egg fusion and male fertility. Functional impairments of acrosome biogenesis are associated with globozoospermia. Acrosome biogenesis is an important aspect of mammalian spermatogenesis, and it involves multiple cellular processes, such as vesicular trafficking, fusion, anchoring of the acrosome to the nucleus and morphogenesis of the acrosome. Although the process of biogenesis of the acrosome has been well documented, the detailed molecular mechanisms remain unclear. Recently, several molecular components were found to contribute to acrosome biogenesis. In this review, the authors summarize the progress that has been made in understanding the molecular mechanisms underlying acrosome biogenesis, and the authors discuss the potential directions of future investigations of this process.

Chapter 2 – Spermatogenesis is a continuous and organized process that occurs throughout the adult life of a male, by which spermatogonia proceed through mitosis, meiosis and complex cytological transformations resulting in the formation of spermatozoa. This process requires precise and highly ordered regulation of gene expression at both the transcriptional and posttranscriptional levels. Recent advances in genome-wide analyses of the mammalian transcriptome have revealed that in addition to mRNAs, several types of noncoding RNAs (ncRNAs), including microRNAs (miRNAs), endogenous small-interfering RNAs (endo-siRNAs), PIWI-interacting RNAs (piRNAs) and long noncoding RNAs (lncRNAs), are extensively transcribed during testis development and spermatogenesis. These ncRNAs are expressed in a cell-specific and step-specific manner to participate in the control of germ cell differentiation during spermatogenesis. In this review, the authors first briefly address the basics of spermatogenesis and the synthesis of ncRNAs, and then they discuss the recent progress in understanding of the functions of miRNAs, endo-siRNAs, piRNAs and lncRNAs in the regulation of spermatogenesis.

Chapter 3 – The mammalian testis has a special immune microenvironment essential for spermatogenesis. The testis is a remarkable immunoprivileged tissue that protects male germ cells from detrimental immune responses. Various immune cells reside in the testis and are able to regulate spermatogenesis. Numerous immunoregulatory cytokines are produced by testicular cells, and they participate in the regulation of testicular immunoprivileged environment. To overcome the immunoprivileged status and enable effective local defense against microbial infections, most testicular cells adopt the innate immune functions. Therefore, a density of local immunoregulatory networks interplay in maintaining testicular immune homeostasis. Disruption of the testicular immune homeostasis may result in orchitis, leading to male infertility. In this article, a review of the current literature on testicular immunoregulation and its underlying mechanisms, along with its effect on testicular functions, is provided.

In: Spermatogenesis
Editor: Gladys Robinson

ISBN: 978-1-63484-715-5

Chapter 1

THE MOLECULAR MECHANISMS UNDERLYING ACROSOME BIOGENESIS

***Chao Liu*[1,2] *and Wei Li*[1,2,*]**

[1]State Key Laboratory of Stem Cell and Reproductive Biology, Institute of Zoology, Chinese Academy of Sciences, Beijing, P.R. China
[2]University of Chinese Academy of Sciences, Beijing, P.R. China

ABSTRACT

The acrosome is a secretory vesicle that covers the anterior part of the sperm nucleus and is essential for sperm-egg fusion and male fertility. Functional impairments of acrosome biogenesis are associated with globozoospermia. Acrosome biogenesis is an important aspect of mammalian spermatogenesis, and it involves multiple cellular processes, such as vesicular trafficking, fusion, anchoring of the acrosome to the nucleus and morphogenesis of the acrosome. Although the process of biogenesis of the acrosome has been well documented, the detailed molecular mechanisms remain unclear. Recently, several molecular components were found to contribute to acrosome biogenesis. In this review, we summarize the progress that has been made in understanding the molecular mechanisms underlying acrosome biogenesis, and we discuss the potential directions of future investigations of this process.

[*] Corresponding author: Dr. Wei Li, Institute of Zoology, Chinese Academy of Sciences, 1 Beichen West Road, Chaoyang District, Beijing 100101, P.R. China. Phone: +86-10-64807529, e-mail: leways@ioz.ac.cn, tel.: 86-10-64807529.

INTRODUCTION

Spermatogenesis is a tightly regulated cellular renovation and differentiation process. It consists of self-renewal and differentiation of spermatogonial stem cells (SSCs), spermatocytic meiosis and spermiogenesis; each of these processes is essential to the continuous, successful production of male gametes [1, 2]. During spermiogenesis, haploid spermatids undergo extensive cellular, molecular and morphological changes, including acrosome biogenesis, flagellum development, cytoplasmic reorganization and chromatin condensation. These changes ultimately result in mature spermatozoa with an acrosome-covered head and motile tail [3-9]. The acrosome is a specialized membranous organelle located over the anterior part of the sperm nucleus that plays an important role in successful fertilization by secreting hydrolytic enzymes to allow the sperm to disperse cumulus cells and/or cross the zona pellucida of the oocyte to form the zygote [10-12]. The absence of acrosomes commonly leads to male infertility, which is related to globozoospermia, an inherited infertility syndrome in humans [13-15].

Acrosome biogenesis is a key event of spermatid differentiation. It develops through the following four major phases: Golgi phase, cap phase, acrosome phase and maturation phase [9, 16, 17]. During the Golgi phase, numerous proacrosomal granules are formed from the edge of the *trans*-Golgi stacks, and then they are transported to the concave region of the nuclear surface and fuse with each other to form a single large acrosomal granule that associates with the nuclear envelope. In the subsequent cap phase, additional proacrosomal granules fuse with the growing acrosome to increase its size, and the latter spread over the anterior nuclear pole like a cap. Then, the acrosome changes its morphology along with the shaping of the sperm nucleus to reach its final shape during the acrosome and maturation phases [9, 16-19]. Although the morphogenetic changes during acrosome biogenesis have been examined extensively and have been well-documented over the past sixty years, the precise molecular mechanisms underlying this process remain unclear. Recently, many acrosome-deficient animal models have been reported (Table 1), and a large number of molecular components have been found to participate in the process of acrosome biogenesis. This review discusses the molecular mechanisms underlying acrosome biogenesis as well as the potential future directions of this field.

Table 1. Mouse models with abnormality of acrosome biogenesis

Gene	Function	Acrosome morphology	Reference
Vesicular trafficking			
Atg7	The E1-like enzyme in autophagy to activate LC3, proacrosomal vesicles trafficking	Fragmented	(Wang et al., 2014)
Fads2	delta-6 desaturase and involved in unsaturated fatty acid metabolism and fusion of proacrosomal vesicles	Fragmented or absent	(Nakamura and Nara, 2004)
Galnt3	GalNAc transferase family protein and initiates the mucin-type O-glycosylation and fusion of proacrosomal vesicles	Absent	(Miyazaki et al., 2013)
Golga3^{repro27}	Golgin family protein, Golgi complex positioning and cargo trafficking	Present and irregular	(Bentson et al., 2013)
Gopc	Proacrosomal vesicle trafficking and fusion	Fragmented	(Yao et al., 2002)
Hook1	Interacts with microtubule and cargo-tethering protein involved in vesicle trafficking	Fragmented	(Moreno et al., 2006)
Hrb	Docking or fusion of Golgi-derived proacrosomal vesicles	Absent	(Kang-Decker et al., 2001)
Ica1l	BAR-domain binding partner of PICK1, Proacrosomal vesicle trafficking	Partially present fragmented	(He et al., 2015)
Ica69/Ica1l	BAR-domain binding partner of PICK1 Proacrosomal vesicles trafficking	Fragmented or absent	(He et al., 2015)
Ift88	Component of the kinesin-2 motor protein Vesicle trafficking	Present and distorted	(Kierszenbaum et al., 2011)
p125	iPLA1family protein and involved in protein secretion from ER via COPII coated vesicle	Absent	(Arimitsu et al., 2011)
Pick1	BAR domain-containing protein and interacts with GOPC, Proacrosomal vesicle trafficking	Fragmented	(Xiao et al., 2009)
Tmf1	Golgi-associated protein, Proacrosomal vesicle trafficking of fusion	Absent	(Lerer-Goldshtein et al., 2010)
Vps54	Retrograde vesicular trafficking from endosomes to the TGN	Absent	(Paiardi et al., 2011)
Anchoring of the acrosome to the nucleus			
Dpy19l2	Inner nuclear membrane protein	Absent	(Pierre et al., 2012)
Spaca1	Acrosomal membrane protein	Partially present Detachment of acrosome from the nucleus	(Fujihara et al., 2012)
Zpbp1	Inner acrosomal membrane protein, binding and penetration into the zona pellucida	Bulged and fragmented	(Lin et al., 2007)
Other			
Csnk2a2	Casein kinase II alpha catalytic subunit, Cyclic-AMP and calcium-independent serine-threonine kinase	Disordered Detachment of acrosome from the nucleus	(Xu et al., 1999)
Gba2	Glucocerebrosidase, hydrolyzes glucosylceramide	Partially present disordered	(Yildiz et al., 2006)
Hsp90b1	ER chaperone, protein folding	Partially present disordered	(Audouard and Christians, 2011)

1. Acrosomal Protein Synthesis and Modification

The endoplasmic reticulum (ER) is the major organelle for protein synthesis and folding [20]. The synthesis of acrosomal proteins, such as acrosin, begins at the pachytene spermatocyte stage and continues throughout the round and elongating spermatid stages [21-23]. These proteins follow the exocytic pathway and are packed in electron-dense core vesicles called proacrosomal granules. Ultrastructural studies have shown that proacrosomal granules also appear at the pachytene stage [22, 24-27]. Many ER-localized proteins have been reported to be detected in the acrosome, such as POMT1 [28], POMT2 [29] and Calreticulin [30]. However, very little data exist regarding the role of the ER in acrosome biogenesis. Hsp90b1 (gp96 or Grp94; glucose-related protein 94), a member of the heat shock protein 90 (Hsp90) family, is found in the ER and is detected in mouse testes [31, 32]. The germ cell conditional knockout of *Hsp90b1* showed deficient spermatozoa with large and globular/abnormal heads, a phenotype reminiscent of human globozoospermia [33]. These findings indicate that Hsp90b1 might be the testis-specific chaperone for the proper folding of acrosomal proteins, and acrosomal protein folding in the ER is important for acrosome biogenesis. β-Glucosidase 2 (GBA2) is a glucocerebrosidase that resides in the ER, and it plays a role in the metabolism of bile acid–glucose conjugates [34]. The disruption of GBA2 produces spermatozoa with distended round heads without an obvious acrosome [35].

2. The Vesicular Trafficking of Acrosomal Granules during Acrosome Biogenesis

After synthesis and proper folding, acrosomal proteins are transported to the concave region of the nuclear surface though acrosomal vesicles, and they fuse with each other to form the acrosome (Figure 1) [9]. There are at least two sources of vesicular transport during acrosome biogenesis, one is derived from the Golgi in the ER–Golgi–acrosome direction and the other is derived from the plasma membrane through endocytosis [9, 19, 36, 37].

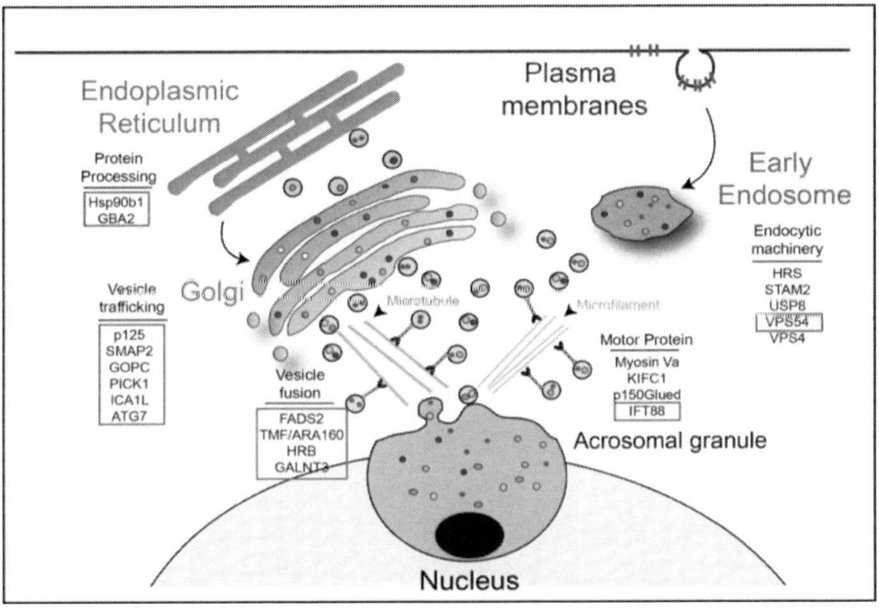

Figure 1. Schematic representation of proacrosomal granule transportation in acrosome biogenesis. After protein processing within the ER, acrosomal proteins are transported to the concave region of the nuclear surface forming the acrosome via two approaches, one from the Golgi in the ER–Golgi–acrosome direction, and the other from the plasma membranes through endocytosis. The proacrosomal granule transportation can be roughly divided into three steps: proacrosomal vesicle formation, trafficking and fusion. The cytoskeleton and its specific molecular motor proteins play key roles in proacrosomal vesicle trafficking. Mice lacking functional copies of the genes highlighted in red boxes display globozoospermia or globozoospermia-like phenotypes.

2.1. ER-Golgi-Acrosome Vesicular Trafficking

2.1.1. Acrosomal Protein Transport from the ER to the Golgi

Many acrosome-located proteins can be transported from the ER through the Golgi to the acrosome [38, 39]. COPII-coated vesicles are involved in the ER-Golgi transportation [40], and they consist of at least two functional parts: the inner layer, which is characterized by the GTPase SAR1 binding to SEC23–SEC24 and selecting specific cargo for packaging into ER-derived transport vesicles, and the outer layer, which is characterized by SEC13–SEC31 deforming the ER membranes to drive the formation of transport vesicles [41]. P125/SEC23ip is a member of the intracellular phospholipase

A1 (iPLA1) family. P125/SEC23ip interacts with both SEC23 and SEC31 to facilitate acrosomal protein transport from the ER to the Golgi. The knockout of *p125* leads to round head spermatozoa without acrosomes, suggesting the importance of the ER transport system in acrosome biogenesis [42-44].

2.1.2. Golgi-Derived Vesicular Trafficking

Acrosome formation is initiated by the budding of proacrosomal vesicles from the Trans Golgi Network (TGN). There is a close relationship between the formation of acrosomal vesicles and the Golgi apparatus [9, 45]. Many Golgi proteins, such as giantin, β-COP, Golgin-97 and Golgin-95/GM130, are detected in the membranes surrounding the acrosome in early stages of spermiogenesis, and they are transported into the Golgi apparatus during the maturation stages [9, 45-47]. β-COP and clathrin-coated vesicles are involved in the anterograde and retrograde transport processes of active Golgi-derived vesicles during acrosome biogenesis [45, 47, 48]. Many classical vesicle trafficking-related proteins are also localized around the acrosomal region [47]. Collectively, these findings indicate that there is highly dynamic Golgi-derived vesicle trafficking during acrosome biogenesis, which can be roughly divided into three steps: the proacrosomal vesicle formation, vesicular trafficking and fusion.

Clathrin and the clathrin assembly protein (CALM) are found to be involved in TGN vesicle formation and transport [49, 50]. The Arf GTPase-activating protein (Arf GAP) activates Arf, which belongs to a family of small GTPases, to regulate the formation of clathrin-coated vesicles [51, 52]. SMAP2 is an Arf GAP protein that binds to CALM and plays multiple roles in various intracellular vesicular trafficking pathways [53, 54]. During acrosome biogenesis, SMAP2 interacts with CALM and syntaxin2, a component of the soluble N-ethylmaleimide–sensitive factor attachment protein receptor (SNARE) complex, to regulate the formation of clathrin-coated vesicles from the TGN and participates in acrosome biogenesis [55].

Some molecular components have been identified during the Golgi-derived vesicular trafficking of acrosome biogenesis. The Golgi-associated PDZ- and coiled-coil motif-containing protein (GOPC) is isolated as a Frizzled-interacting protein and plays a role in vesicular transport from the Golgi apparatus to the plasma membrane [56]. GOPC is predominantly localized at the Trans Golgi region in round spermatids and is required for proacrosomal vesicle transport and fusion with the growing acrosomal cap [57]. GOLGA3 is a 170 kDa Golgi-associated protein that is highly expressed in the Golgi apparatus of round spermatids. GOLGA3 may participate in acrosome biogenesis through binding with GOPC [58-60]. Protein interacting with C kinase 1 (PICK1) is a Bin-Amphiphysin-Rvs (BAR) domain-containing protein that promotes the curvature and scission of membranes during budding and participates in protein trafficking [61]. PICK1 is localized around the Golgi apparatus in spermatids. It interacts with GOPC to facilitate the formation of trafficking vesicles from the Golgi apparatus and transportation to the acrosome [62]. ICA1L was identified as a new BAR-domain binding partner of PICK1 that is trafficked together with PICK1 at different stages of spermiogenesis. *ICA1L*-knockout mice also exhibited abnormalities in acrosome formation [63]. Macroautophagy (hereafter referred to as autophagy) is the primary intracellular catabolic mechanism for degrading and recycling long-lived proteins and organelles by a double-membrane vesicle, the autophagosome [64, 65]. The autophagy machinery is also required for acrosomal vesicular trafficking during acrosome biogenesis. LC3 is activated by ATG7 and then transferred to the Golgi-derived vesicles either directly or indirectly by phagophore-like structures, finally inducing the fusion of those vesicles with each other or facilitating their transport to the nucleus-associated acrosome [66]. Some other Golgi-derived vesicular trafficking-related proteins have been reported to be localized around the Golgi apparatus in spermatids, such as MgcRabGAP [67], Rab6 [68], and NYD-SP12 [69]; however, understanding their precise molecular roles during acrosome biogenesis will require further investigation.

After being transported to the nuclear surface, acrosomal granules fuse with each other to form a single large acrosomal granule. Vesicle fusion relies on the formation of a SNARE complex consisting of syntaxin, soluble NSF attachment protein (SNAP), and vesicle-associated membrane protein (VAMP), which drive the union of opposing membranes [70-72]. These components and their related proteins, such as syntaxin 1, syntaxin 2, VAD1. 3/AEP1 and VAD1.2/AEP2, were detected around the acrosomal region in spermatids [27, 73-75]. Free polyunsaturated fatty acids (PUFAs), including arachidonic acid (AA) and docosahexaenoic acid (DHA), can activate syntaxin to form a binary SNARE complex and promote vesicle fusion [72, 76]. The fatty acid desaturase 2 (FADS2), also known as a delta-6 desaturase, catalyzes the first step of the synthesis of highly unsaturated fatty acids (HUFAs) as well as the last desaturation step of DHA [77]. The disruption of FADS2 leads to scattered syntaxin 2 in reticular structures and impaired proacrosomal vesicles fusion, which results in the absence of acrosome formation [78]. TMF/ARA160 is a Golgi-associated protein that is involved in vesicle tethering to target membranes [79, 80]. The disruption of TMF/ARA160 results in spermatozoa without acrosomes, suggesting that TMF/ARA160 is required for the transport and docking of proacrosomal vesicles to the apical nuclear surface [81]. HRB is a protein that contains several NPF motifs (Asn-Pro-Phe) and interacts with proteins with EPS15 homology domains [82]. HRB binds to the cytosolic surface of proacrosomal transporting vesicles and exists between the Golgi apparatus and the nuclear surface, which is regarded as critical for the docking or fusion of Golgi-derived proacrosomal vesicles [83]. Polypeptide N-acetylgalactosaminyl-transferase 3 (GALNT3) is a member of the GalNAc transferase family that is involved in the initiation of mucin-type O-glycosylation [84]. GALNT3 is localized in the cis-medial parts of the Golgi stacks of spermatocytes and spermatids. The disruption of GALNT3 results in proacrosomal vesicles failing to fuse and being present on the nuclear envelope, indicating the importance of protein O-glycosylation in the fusion of proacrosomal vesicles [85]. Many vesicle formation or trafficking-related proteins, such as SMAP2 and GOPC also participate in proacrosomal vesicle fusion [55, 57].

2.2. Endocytic Vesicular Trafficking

In addition to Golgi-derived vesicular trafficking, components of the endocytic machinery and plasma membranes are also involved in the biogenesis of the acrosome [9, 19, 86, 87]. In 1996, West and Willison treated cultured germ cells with a Golgi apparatus inhibitor, Brefeldin A, and found that the Golgi was disrupted but not the acrosome [36]. A novel membrane protein, acrosome formation-associated factor (AFAF), was detected in the EEA1-positive early endosomes (EEs) and in the inner and outer membranes of the forming acrosome in spermatids [88]. These results indicate that early endosomes and the plasma membrane may also be directly involved in acrosome biogenesis. Much of the endocytic machinery and its related proteins were detected during acrosome biogenesis, including the Endosomal Sorting Complex Required for Transport-0 (ESCRT-0), EEA1 [89], SH3P13 [90], DYDC1 [91], and GLUT8 [92, 93]. In the initiation of endocytosis, ubiquitination serves as a sorting signal on protein cargo, and the ESCRT-0 complex, HRS and STAM2, recognize and bind to ubiquitinated cargo through their ubiquitin-interacting motifs to internalize targeted cargo into the endocytic pathway [94]. During acrosome biogenesis, a deubiquitinating enzyme, ubiquitin-specific peptidase 8 (USP8), interacts with STAM2 to regulate endosomal sorting and recruitment targeting to the early endosomes, and these structures finally develop into EEA1-positive acrosomes [89, 95, 96]. VPS54 is a component of the Golgi Associated Retrograde Protein (GARP) complex and is involved in retrograde vesicular trafficking from endosomes to the TGN [97, 98]. VPS54 co-localizes with the developing acrosome in spermatids, and missense mutations of VPS54 (L967Q) in *wobbler* mice prevent the formation of acrosomes. Additionally, USP8 positive endosomes remain single and scattered vesicles do not contribute to acrosome formation in the presence of missense mutations of VPS54 (L967Q) in *wobbler* mice, indicating the importance of endocytosis in acrosome biogenesis [89, 99]. Vesicle-associated membrane protein 4 (VAMP4) is a v-SNARE protein that also participates in retrograde trafficking from the early endosome to the TGN [100]. Knockdown of VAMP4 causes defects in acrosomal vesicle fusion and subsequent acrosome formation [101].

2.3. Cytoskeletal Transportation during Acrosome Biogenesis

Cytoskeletons and their specific molecular motor proteins are known to play key roles in organelle and membrane-bound vesicle transportation in somatic cells, including Golgi-derived secretory granules [102-105]. During acrosome biogenesis, acrosomal vesicular trafficking also utilizes F-actin, microtubules and their related motor proteins [106].

In the F-actin route, the actin-based motor Myosin Va and its receptor, RAB 27a/b, are present in the Golgi and Golgi-derived proacrosomal vesicles of spermatids [107, 108]. In the microtubule route, microtubule-associated kinesin and dynein motors and non-motor proteins have been shown to participate in cargo trafficking at the Golgi and from the Golgi to the acrosome [106]. The disruption of microtubules via colchicine or nocodazole treatment causes retardation of acrosome formation, and the Golgi apparatus loses its typical membranous stack conformation and disintegrates into numerous small vesicles [109, 110]. Thus, microtubule-dependent trafficking of transport vesicles between the Golgi apparatus and the acrosome might play a vital role in acrosome biogenesis. KIFC1 is a member of the C-terminal class of kinesin-related proteins. KIFC1 first appears around the Golgi apparatus in early spermatids, then redistributes to the acrosomal vesicle [111]. IFT88 is a member of the IFT-B protein complex, which couples with kinesin-2 motor protein to promote the mobilization of cargo along the microtubules of the axoneme [112] and is present in the Golgi-derived proacrosomal vesicles of spermatids [113]. The *Oak Ridge Polycystic Kidney* (*ORPK*) mouse has a hypomorphic mutation in the *Ift88* gene [114], and the deficiency of IFT88 might influence proacrosomal vesicular trafficking and induce abnormalities in acrosome biogenesis [113]. p150Glued is a subunit of dynein that binds to microtubules and enhances the processivity of the dynein motor [115]. p150Glued localizes at the cytosolic side of proacrosomal vesicles in early spermatids, followed by localization to the outer and inner acrosomal membranes [106]. GMAP210 is a Golgi microtubule-associated protein, which contains a GRAB (GRIP-related Arf binding) domain and an ALPS (amphipathic lipid-packing sensor) domain, that binds membranes of spherical and flat curvature with its N- and C-terminal domains [106, 116-118]. GMAP210 resides in the cis-Golgi of spermatids and is involved in proacrosomal vesicle transportation [113] HOOK1 is a member of the Hook family of coiled-coil proteins, which function as microtubule- and cargo-tethering proteins by binding with microtubules and cargo through the N- and C-terminal domains, respectively [119]. In spermatids, HOOK1 was detected in the TGN associated with Golgi-derived proacrosomal vesicles [106]. The *azh* mouse contains a deletion of exons 10 and 11 in the *Hook1* gene [120], leading to the fragmentation of the Golgi apparatus and acrosome [109]. In the acrosome endocytic vesicular trafficking system, USP8-sorted acrosomal vesicle transport is also mediated by microtubules because USP8 is recruited by microtubules [89, 121]. Therefore, acrosomal vesicular trafficking mediated by cytoskeletons and their associated motor and non-motor proteins is a key event in acrosome biogenesis.

3. The Anchoring of the Acrosome to the Nucleus

After being transported to the concave region of the nuclear surface, the acrosome attaches to and spread over the nucleus. An F-actin-keratin 5-containing cytoskeletal plate, the acroplaxome, was found to anchor the developing acrosome to the nuclear envelope [122]. The acroplaxome consists of a marginal ring, and the ring is composed of keratin 5-containing intermediate filaments associated with the leading edge of the inner acrosomal membrane [122]. Thus, the anchoring of the acrosome to the nucleus can be divided into three parts: the acrosome membrane-acroplaxome interface, the acroplaxome and the acroplaxome-nuclear membrane interface (Figure 2).

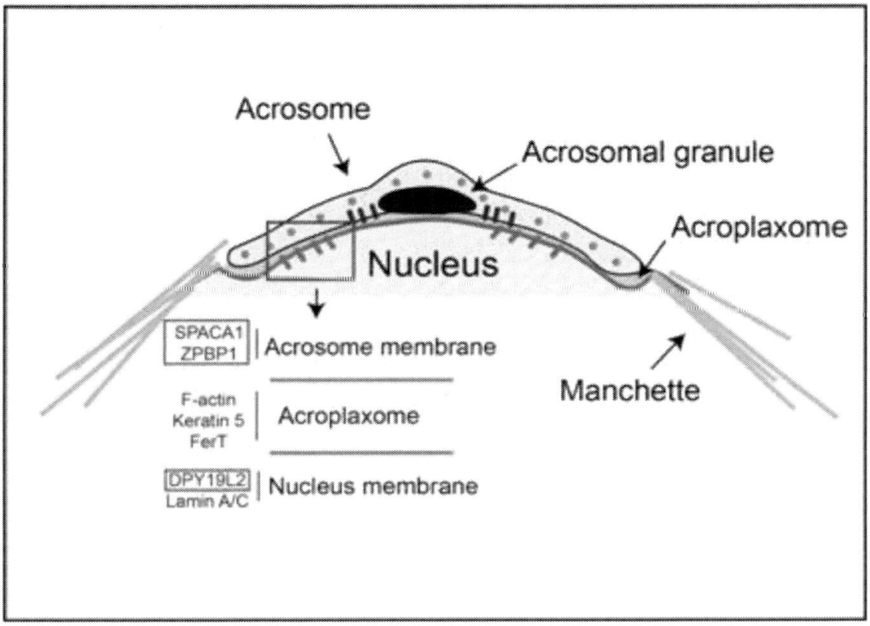

Figure 2. Proteins involved in the anchoring of the acrosome to nucleus. The connection between the acrosome and the nucleus can be divided into three parts: the interaction of the inner acrosomal membrane with the acroplaxome, the acroplaxome, and the interaction of the acroplaxome with the outer and inner nuclear membranes of the nuclear envelope. Mice lacking functional copies of the genes highlighted in red boxes display globozoospermia or globozoospermia-like phenotypes.

Sperm acrosome-associated 1 (SPACA1) is an acrosomal membrane protein, and it is localized exclusively on a peripheral part of the acrosomal membrane forming a ring-like structure in step 7 spermatids. Disruption of SPACA1 impairs the formation of intermediate filament bundles of the acroplaxome, which leads to the detachment of the acrosome from the nucleus and abnormal acrosome formation [123]. Zona pellucida-binding protein 1 (ZPBP1) is an inner acrosomal membrane protein, originally identified in pigs and named for its binding to the oocyte zona pellucid [124, 125]. In the early elongating spermatids, ZPBP1 is localized on the periphery of the acrosomal membrane [125]. The absence of ZPBP1 prevents proper acrosome compaction, resulting in acrosome fragmentation [124]. The protein level of Spaca1 was dramatically reduced in mice with a ZPBP1 disruption, indicating that the acrosome formation defect in *Zpbp1*-disrupted mice might be due to the loss of Spaca1 from their acrosomes [123].

In addition to F-actin and keratin 5, other molecular components were also detected around the acroplaxome, such as Profilin 3 (actin binding protein) [126], Profilin 4 [126, 127], RNF19, PSMC3 [128], and Fyn [129]. Fer Testis (FerT) is a member of the Fes/Fps family of nonreceptor tyrosine kinases. FerT participates in the regulation of cytoskeletal reorganization, cell adhesion, and vesicular transport [130]. The FerT protein is associated with the cytosolic side of the outer acrosome membrane adjacent to the inner acrosome membrane facing the acroplaxome, and it coexists with an F-actin regulator, phosphorylated cortactin, in the acroplaxome [131, 132]. Thus, FerT might participate in F-actin structural changes in the acroplaxome and in the anchoring of the acrosome to the nucleus by regulating the phosphorylation of cortactin. However, the precise molecular mechanism still needs to be further explored.

DPY19L2 is a transmembrane protein with 10 putative transmembrane segments that is located in the inner nuclear membrane (INM) facing the acrosome. DPY19L2 could function as a bridge between the nucleus and the acroplaxome. The absence of DP19L2 leads to the disruption of the layered structure present at the nuclear/acroplaxome junction and detachment of the acrosome and the acroplaxome from the nucleus during acrosome spreading, which results in the loss of the acrosome [133]. Lamin A/C is an A-type lamin that is a major structural component of the nuclear envelope (NE) [134]. Lamin A/C is localized to the acroplaxome from round spermatids to mature spermatozoa in spermiogenesis. Lamin A/C might participate in the connection between the acroplaxome and the nucleus, as it can interact with a microtubule plus-end-tracking protein, CLIP170. Knockdown of Lamin A/C increased the fragmentation of the acrosome and impaired acrosome biogenesis [135].

4. The Morphogenesis of the Acrosome

During the acrosome and maturation phases, the acrosome will change its morphology along with the shaping of the sperm nucleus to reach its final shape [9]. As the acrosome is anchored on the nucleus, the morphological shaping of the acrosome is highly associated with the process of sperm head shaping. Many malformed sperm head animal models also have abnormal acrosomes, and mutations in the first defined sperm head morphogenesis gene, *Csnk2a2*, results in abnormal acrosomes [136]. The acroplaxome, manchette, head-to-tail coupling apparatus in spermatids, apical ectoplasmic specialization (aES), and apical tubulobulbar complex (aTBC) in Sertoli cells are the major devices which are involved in acrosome shaping [137-139].

The acrosome is localized on F-actin-based acroplaxomes attached to the spermatid nuclear envelope. The manchette, consisting of a perinuclear rings with inserted microtubules, lies subjacent to the marginal ring of the acroplaxome with a narrow gap. In head-to-tail coupling, the sperm tail axoneme initiates its assembly from the centrosomal region located at the pole opposite of the acrosome. The apical ectoplasmic specialization of Sertoli cells mechanically grasps the head of spermatids with bundles of actin filaments, forming a stack of hoops embracing the acrosomal region of the elongating spermatid [137, 138, 140]. During acrosome shaping, all of these cytoskeleton-based processes may provide the major impetus to drive and support the morphological changes. The apical tubulobulbar complex, composed of fine filaments of actin surrounded by a tubular portion and a double plasma membrane bulbous portion flanked by smooth endoplasmic reticulum in the Sertoli-germ cell interface, might eliminate excess acrosomal content via the phagocytes of Sertoli cells, leading to the shaping of the spermatid acrosome prior to sperm release [139, 141]. Many molecular components participate in these acrosome shaping processes; however, the detailed mechanisms are still not yet fully understood [137, 138].

5. The Acrosome, Modified Lysosome or Autolysosome?

Because it shares some common features with lysosomes, such as low internal acidic pH and the presence of lysosomal enzymes, the acrosome has been postulated to be a modified lysosome [142]. However, as described above, the acrosome cannot be considered as a canonical lysosome because both the endocytic pathway and the biosynthetic pathway are involved in acrosome biogenesis. Usually, the biogenesis of lysosome-related organelles (LROs) require the above two pathways, so the acrosome may be a novel LRO [19, 66, 89]. Although restricted to certain specialized cell types, LROs represent a family of membrane-enclosed organelles, which includes melanosomes, lytic granules, platelet dense bodies, exosomes and synaptosomes [19, 143, 144]. LROs are a heterogeneous group of vesicles that share features with lysosomes but have distinct morphology, composition and/or function [143, 145]. In contrast to classical secretory granules, which are generated directly from the TGN, the early endosome is the crucial protein-sorting hub of LRO biogenesis [145]. In fact, approximately thirty years ago, two sources of vesicular transport to the acrosome were identified using two fluorescent lipid compounds labeling the Golgi and endocytic vesicles [87]. The endocytic machinery was found to participate in acrosome biogenesis. Recently, the autophagy machinery has also been identified as required for acrosomal vesicular trafficking during acrosome biogenesis, which suggests that the acrosome, or even all of the LROs, may originate from an autolysosome rather than a lysosome alone [66].

Conclusion and Future Perspectives

Abnormal acrosome biogenesis often leads to globozoospermia in humans, and many acrosome biogenesis-related genes are mutated in globozoospermia patients, including SPATA16, PICK1 and DPY19L2 [146]. Although substantial important progress in this field has been made, defining the cellular and molecular mechanisms underlying acrosome biogenesis remains a difficult task. With the development of new mass spectrometry and genome editing techniques, the study of acrosome biogenesis may enter a new explosive developmental era. Isolation, purification, and subsequent analysis by mass spectrometry of the acrosomal vesicles or acrosomes from different developmental stages during spermatogenesis may represent a powerful strategy for the identification of acrosome-specific components. With the maturation of the CRISPR/Cas9 system, the core acrosome biogenesis components may be screened from more knockout animal models. In addition to the classical vesicular trafficking machinery, the identification of some new tissue-specific molecular components that participate in acrosomal vesicle transport, such as some specific trafficking factors, motor proteins or intermediate proteins between the Golgi and endocytosis, is highly anticipated. Such information will greatly deepen our understanding of the precise molecular mechanisms underlying acrosome biogenesis. The development of new visible markers for different stages of acrosomal granules/vesicles or acrosomes is urgently needed for the study of acrosome biogenesis. Because acrosome biogenesis often lasts for more than 20 days [9], it is difficult to detect this dynamic process under physiological conditions. The development of new *in vitro* germ cells or methods of culturing seminiferous tubules should help us monitor this process by examining the transport of labeled acrosomal cargo. The factors that initiate acrosome biogenesis are still completely unknown, and some cellular signals, transcription factors or even hormonal regulation may participate in this process. By addressing these open questions and aiming future studies in the above mentioned directions, we will greatly broaden our knowledge of acrosome biogenesis, thus providing potential new therapeutic targets for globozoospermia and new methods of contraception in the future.

REFERENCES

[1] Hess, R. A., Renato de Franca, L. Spermatogenesis and cycle of the seminiferous epithelium. *Advances in experimental medicine and biology* 2008; 636:1-15.

[2] Roosen-Runge, E. C. The process of spermatogenesis in mammals. *Biological reviews of the Cambridge Philosophical Society* 1962; 37: 343-77.

[3] Fabian, L., Brill, J. A. Drosophila spermiogenesis: Big things come from little packages. *Spermatogenesis* 2012; 2:197-212.

[4] Toshimori, K., Ito, C. Formation and organization of the mammalian sperm head. *Archives of histology and cytology* 2003; 66:383-96.

[5] Rathke, C., Baarends, W. M., Awe, S., Renkawitz-Pohl, R. Chromatin dynamics during spermiogenesis. *Biochimica et biophysica acta* 2014; 1839:155-68.

[6] Oko, R., Sutovsky, P. Biogenesis of sperm perinuclear theca and its role in sperm functional competence and fertilization. *Journal of reproductive immunology* 2009; 83:2-7.

[7] Dadoune, J. P. The cellular biology of mammalian spermatids: a review. *Bulletin de l'Association des anatomistes* 1994; 78:33-40.

[8] Hermo, L., Pelletier, R. M., Cyr, D. G., Smith, C. E. Surfing the wave, cycle, life history, and genes/proteins expressed by testicular germ cells. Part 1: background to spermatogenesis, spermatogonia, and spermatocytes. *Microscopy research and technique* 2010; 73:241-78.

[9] Hermo, L., Pelletier, R. M., Cyr, D. G., Smith, C. E. Surfing the wave, cycle, life history, and genes/proteins expressed by testicular germ cells. Part 2: changes in spermatid organelles associated with development of spermatozoa. *Microscopy research and technique* 2010; 73:279-319.

[10] Barros, C., Crosby, J. A., Moreno, R. D. Early steps of sperm-egg interactions during mammalian fertilization. *Cell biology international* 1996; 20:33-9.

[11] Tulsiani, D. R., Abou-Haila, A., Loeser, C. R., Pereira, B. M. The biological and functional significance of the sperm acrosome and acrosomal enzymes in mammalian fertilization. *Experimental cell research* 1998; 240:151-64.

[12] Tulsiani, D. R., Yoshida-Komiya, H., Araki, Y. Mammalian fertilization: a carbohydrate-mediated event. *Biology of reproduction* 1997; 57:487-94.

[13] Anton-Lamprecht, I., Kotzur, B., Schopf, E. Round-headed human spermatozoa. *Fertil. Steril.* 1976; 27:685-93.

[14] Lalonde, L., Langlais, J., Antaki, P., Chapdelaine, A., Roberts, K. D., Bleau, G. Male infertility associated with round-headed acrosomeless spermatozoa. *Fertil. Steril.* 1988; 49:316-21.

[15] Schill, W. B. Some Disturbances of Acrosomal Development and Function in Human Spermatozoa. *Hum. Reprod.* 1991; 6:969-78.

[16] Clermont, Y., Leblond, C. P. Spermiogenesis of Man, Monkey, Ram and Other Mammals as Shown by the Periodic Acid-Schiff Technique. *American Journal of Anatomy* 1955; 96:229-53.

[17] Abou-Haila, A., Tulsiani, D. R. Mammalian sperm acrosome: formation, contents, and function. *Archives of biochemistry and biophysics* 2000; 379:173-82.

[18] Leblond, C. P., Clermont, Y. Spermiogenesis of Rat, Mouse, Hamster and Guinea Pig as Revealed by the Periodic Acid-Fuchsin Sulfurous Acid Technique. *American Journal of Anatomy* 1952; 90:167-215.

[19] Berruti, G., Paiardi, C. Acrosome biogenesis: Revisiting old questions to yield new insights. *Spermatogenesis* 2011; 1:95-8.

[20] Vitale, A., Ceriotti, A., Denecke, J. The Role of the Endoplasmic-Reticulum in Protein-Synthesis, Modification and Intracellular-Transport. *J. Exp. Bot.* 1993; 44:1417-44.

[21] Kashiwabara, S., Arai, Y., Kodaira, K., Baba, T. Acrosin Biosynthesis in Meiotic and Postmeiotic Spermatogenic Cells. *Biochem. Bioph. Res. Co.* 1990; 173:240-5.

[22] Anakwe, O. O., Gerton, G. L. Acrosome Biogenesis Begins during Meiosis - Evidence from the Synthesis and Distribution of an Acrosomal Glycoprotein, Acrogranin, during Guinea-Pig Spermatogenesis. *Biology of reproduction* 1990; 42:317-28.

[23] Escalier, D., Gallo, J. M., Albert, M., Meduri, G., Bermudez, D., David, G., Schrevel, J. Human Acrosome Biogenesis - Immunodetection of Proacrosin in Primary Spermatocytes and of Its Partitioning Pattern during Meiosis. *Development* 1991; 113:779-88.

[24] Suarezquian, C. A., An, Q., Jelesoff, N., Dym, M. The Golgi-Apparatus of Rat Pachytene Spermatocytes during Spermatogenesis. *Anat. Rec.* 1991; 229:16-26.

[25] Fawcett, D. W. Gametogenesis in the male: prospects for its control. The symposium/*The Society for Developmental Biology Society for Developmental Biology Symposium* 1975:25-53.

[26] Nicander, L., Ploen, L. Fine structure of spermatogonia and primary spermatocytes in rabbits. *Zeitschrift fur Zellforschung und mikroskopische Anatomie* 1969; 99:221-34.

[27] Ramalho-Santos, J., Schatten, G., Moreno, R. D. Control of membrane fusion during spermiogenesis and the acrosome reaction. *Biology of reproduction* 2002; 67:1043-51.

[28] Prados, B., Pena, A., Cotarelo, R. P., Valero, M. C., Cruces, J. Expression of the murine Pomt1 gene in both the developing brain and adult muscle tissues and its relationship with clinical aspects of Walker-Warburg syndrome. *Am. J. Pathol.* 2007; 170:1659-68.

[29] Willer, T., Amselgruber, W., Deutzmann, R., Strahl, S. Characterization of POMT2, a novel member of the PMT protein O-mannosyltransferase family specifically localized to the acrosome of mammalian spermatids. *Glycobiology* 2002; 12:771-83.

[30] Nakamura, M., Moriya, M., Baba, T., Michikawa, Y., Yamanobe, T., Arai, K., Okinaga, S., Kobayashi, T. An Endoplasmic-Reticulum Protein, Calreticulin, Is Transported into the Acrosome of Rat Sperm. *Experimental cell research* 1993; 205:101-10.

[31] Asquith, K. L., Harman, A. J., McLaughlin, E. A., Nixon, B., Aitken, R. J. Localization and significance of molecular chaperones, heat shock protein 1, and tumor rejection antigen gp96 in the male reproductive tract and during capacitation and acrosome reaction. *Biology of reproduction* 2005; 72:328-37.

[32] Yang, Y., Li, Z. Roles of heat shock protein gp96 in the ER quality control: redundant or unique function? *Molecules and cells* 2005; 20: 173-82.

[33] Audouard, C., Christians, E. Hsp90b1 knockout targeted to male germline: a mouse model for globozoospermia. *Fertil. Steril.* 2011; 95: 1475-U326.

[34] Matern, H., Heinemann, H., Legler, G., Matern, S. Purification and characterization of a microsomal bile acid beta-glucosidase from human liver. *The Journal of biological chemistry* 1997; 272:11261-7.

[35] Yildiz, Y., Matern, H., Thompson, B., Allegood, J. C., Warren, R. L., Ramirez, D. M., Hammer, R. E., Hamra, F. K., Matern, S., Russell, D. W. Mutation of beta-glucosidase 2 causes glycolipid storage disease and impaired male fertility. *The Journal of clinical investigation* 2006; 116: 2985-94.

[36] West, A. P., Willison, K. R. Brefeldin A and mannose 6-phosphate regulation of acrosomic related vesicular trafficking. *European journal of cell biology* 1996; 70:315-21.

[37] Tanii, I., Toshimori, K., Araki, S., Oura, C. Extra-Golgi pathway of an acrosomal antigen during spermiogenesis in the rat. *Cell and tissue research* 1992; 270:451-7.

[38] Cotman, M., Jezek, D., Fon Tacer, K., Frangez, R., Rozman, D. A functional cytochrome P450 lanosterol 14 alpha-demethylase CYP51 enzyme in the acrosome: transport through the Golgi and synthesis of meiosis-activating sterols. *Endocrinology* 2004; 145:1419-26.

[39] Nakamura, M., Moriya, M., Baba, T., Michikawa, Y., Yamanobe, T., Arai, K., Okinaga, S., Kobayashi, T. An endoplasmic reticulum protein, calreticulin, is transported into the acrosome of rat sperm. *Experimental cell research* 1993; 205:101-10.

[40] Jensen, D., Schekman, R. COPII-mediated vesicle formation at a glance. *Journal of cell science* 2011; 124:1-4.

[41] Brandizzi, F., Barlowe, C. Organization of the ER-Golgi interface for membrane traffic control. *Nature reviews Molecular cell biology* 2013; 14:382-92.

[42] Tani, K., Mizoguchi, T., Iwamatsu, A., Hatsuzawa, K., Tagaya, M. P125 is a novel mammalian Sec23p-interacting protein with structural similarity to phospholipid-modifying proteins. *J. Biol. Chem.* 1999; 274: 20505-12.

[43] Ong, Y. S., Tang, B. L., Loo, L. S., Hong, W. J. p125A exists as part of the mammalian Sec13/Sec31 COPII subcomplex to facilitate ER-Golgi transport. *Journal of Cell Biology* 2010; 190:331-45.

[44] Arimitsu, N., Kogure, T., Baba, T., Nakao, K., Hamamoto, H., Sekimizu, K., Yamamoto, A., Nakanishi, H., Taguchi, R., Tagaya, M. et al. p125/Sec23-interacting protein (Sec23ip) is required for spermiogenesis. *Febs Lett.* 2011; 585:2171-6.

[45] Moreno, R. D., Ramalho-Santos, J., Sutovsky, P., Chan, E. K., Schatten, G. Vesicular traffic and golgi apparatus dynamics during mammalian spermatogenesis: implications for acrosome architecture. *Biology of reproduction* 2000; 63:89-98.

[46] Moreno, R. D., Ramalho-Santos, J., Chan, E. K., Wessel, G. M., Schatten, G. The Golgi apparatus segregates from the lysosomal/acrosomal vesicle during rhesus spermiogenesis: structural alterations. *Developmental biology* 2000; 219:334-49.

[47] Ramalho-Santos, J., Moreno, R. D., Wessel, G. M., Chan, E. K., Schatten, G. Membrane trafficking machinery components associated with the mammalian acrosome during spermiogenesis. *Experimental cell research* 2001; 267:45-60.

[48] Martinez-Menarguez, J. A., Geuze, H. J., Ballesta, J. Identification of two types of beta-COP vesicles in the Golgi complex of rat spermatids. *European journal of cell biology* 1996; 71:137-43.

[49] Bonifacino, J. S., Glick, B. S. The mechanisms of vesicle budding and fusion. *Cell* 2004; 116:153-66.

[50] Robinson, D. G., Pimpl, P. Clathrin and post-Golgi trafficking: a very complicated issue. *Trends Plant Sci.* 2014; 19:134-9.

[51] D'Souza-Schorey, C., Chavrier, P. ARF proteins: roles in membrane traffic and beyond. *Nat. Rev. Mol. Cell. Bio.* 2006; 7:347-58.

[52] Randazzo, P. A., Hirsch, D. S. Arf GAPs: multifunctional proteins that regulate membrane traffic and actin remodelling. *Cell Signal* 2004; 16: 401-13.

[53] Natsume, W., Tanabe, K., Kon, S., Yoshida, N., Watanabe, T., Torii, T., Satake, M. SMAP2, a novel ARF GTPase-activating protein, interacts with clathrin and clathrin assembly protein and functions on the AP-1-positive early endosome/trans-Golgi network. *Molecular biology of the cell* 2006; 17:2592-603.

[54] Funaki, T., Kon, S., Ronn, R. E., Henmi, Y., Kobayashi, Y., Watanabe, T., Nakayama, K., Tanabe, K., Satake, M. Localization of SMAP2 to the TGN and its function in the regulation of TGN protein transport. *Cell structure and function* 2011; 36:83-95.

[55] Funaki, T., Kon, S., Tanabe, K., Natsume, W., Sato, S., Shimizu, T., Yoshida, N., Wong, W. F., Ogura, A., Ogawa, T. et al. The Arf GAP SMAP2 is necessary for organized vesicle budding from the trans-Golgi network and subsequent acrosome formation in spermiogenesis. *Molecular biology of the cell* 2013; 24:2633-44.

[56] Yao, R., Maeda, T., Takada, S., Noda, T. Identification of a PDZ domain containing Golgi protein, GOPC, as an interaction partner of frizzled. *Biochem. Biophys. Res. Commun.* 2001; 286:771-8.

[57] Yao, R., Ito, C., Natsume, Y., Sugitani, Y., Yamanaka, H., Kuretake, S., Yanagida, K., Sato, A., Toshimori, K., Noda, T. Lack of acrosome

formation in mice lacking a Golgi protein, GOPC. *Proceedings of the National Academy of Sciences of the United States of America* 2002; 99: 11211-6.

[58] Banu, Y., Matsuda, M., Yoshihara, M., Kondo, M., Sutou, S., Matsukuma, S. Golgi matrix protein gene, Golga3/Mea2, rearranged and re-expressed in pachytene spermatocytes restores spermatogenesis in the mouse. *Molecular reproduction and development* 2002; 61:288-301.

[59] Bentson, L. F., Agbor, V. A., Agbor, L. N., Lopez, A. C., Nfonsam, L. E., Bornstein, S. S., Handel, M. A., Linder, C. C. New point mutation in Golga3 causes multiple defects in spermatogenesis. *Andrology-Us* 2013; 1:440-50.

[60] Hicks, S. W., Machamer, C. E. Isoform-specific interaction of golgin-160 with the Golgi-associated protein PIST. *J. Biol. Chem.* 2005; 280: 28944-51.

[61] Arvan, P., Castle, D. Neuroendocrinology: regulated secretory cells go to the BAR for a bud. *Nature reviews Endocrinology* 2013; 9:443-4.

[62] Xiao, N., Kam, C., Shen, C., Jin, W., Wang, J., Lee, K. M., Jiang, L., Xia, J. PICK1 deficiency causes male infertility in mice by disrupting acrosome formation. *The Journal of clinical investigation* 2009; 119: 802-12.

[63] He, J., Xia, M., Tsang, W. H., Chow, K. L., Xia, J. ICA1L forms BAR-domain complexes with PICK1 and is crucial for acrosome formation in spermiogenesis. *Journal of cell science* 2015; 128:3822-36.

[64] Mizushima, N., Levine, B. Autophagy in mammalian development and differentiation. *Nature cell biology* 2010; 12:823-30.

[65] Yang, Z. F., Klionsky, D. J. An Overview of the Molecular Mechanism of Autophagy. *Curr. Top Microbiol.* 2009; 335:1-32.

[66] Wang, H. N., Wan, H. F., Li, X. X., Liu, W. X., Chen, Q., Wang, Y. Q., Yang, L., Tang, H. M., Zhang, X. J., Duan, E. K. et al. Atg7 is required for acrosome biogenesis during spermatogenesis in mice. *Cell Res.* 2014; 24:852-69.

[67] Lin, Y. H., Lin, Y. M., Kuo, Y. C., Wang, Y. Y., Kuo, P. L. Identification and characterization of a novel Rab GTPase-activating protein in spermatids. *Int. J. Androl.* 2011; 34:E358-E67.

[68] Vivero-Salmeron, G., Ballesta, J., Martinez-Menarguez, J. A. Heterotypic tubular connections at the endoplasmic reticulum-Golgi complex interface. *Histochemistry and cell biology* 2008; 130:709-17.

[69] Xu, M., Xiao, J. H., Chen, J., Li, J. M., Yin, L. L., Zhu, H., Zhou, Z. M., Sha, J. H. Identification and characterization of a novel human testis-specific Golgi protein, NYD-SP12. *Mol. Hum. Reprod.* 2003; 9:9-17.

[70] Zhao, M., Brunger, A. T. Recent advances in deciphering the structure and molecular mechanism of the AAA + ATPase N-ethylmaleimide Sensitive Factor (NSF). *Journal of molecular biology* 2015.

[71] Ungermann, C., Langosch, D. Functions of SNAREs in intracellular membrane fusion and lipid bilayer mixing. *Journal of cell science* 2005; 118:3819-28.

[72] Rizo, J., Sudhof, T. C. SNAREs and Munc18 in synaptic vesicle fusion. *Nat. Rev. Neurosci.* 2002; 3:641-53.

[73] Katafuchi, K., Mori, T., Toshimori, K., Iida, H. Localization of a syntaxin isoform, syntaxin 2, to the acrosomal region of rodent spermatozoa. *Molecular reproduction and development* 2000; 57:375-83.

[74] Zuo, Y., Gao, J., Yeung, W. S. B., Lee, K. F. The testis-specific VAD1. 3/AEP1 interacts with beta-actin and syntaxin 1 and directs peri-nuclear/ Golgi expression with bipartite nucleus localization (BNL) sequence. *Biochem. Bioph. Res.* Co 2010; 401:275-80.

[75] Lee, K. F., Tam, Y. T., Zuo, Y., Cheong, A. W., Pang, R. T., Lee, N. P., Shum, C. K., Tam, P. C., Cheung, A. N., Yang, Z. M. et al. Characterization of an acrosome protein VAD1.2/AEP2 which is differentially expressed in spermatogenesis. *Mol. Hum. Reprod.* 2008; 14:465-74.

[76] Rickman, C., Davletov, B. Arachidonic acid allows SNARE complex formation in the presence of Munc18. *Chemistry and biology* 2005; 12: 545-53.

[77] Nakamura, M. T., Nara, T. Y. Structure, function, and dietary regulation of Delta 6, Delta 5, and Delta 9 desaturases. *Annu. Rev. Nutr.* 2004; 24: 345-76.

[78] Roqueta-Rivera, M., Abbott, T. L., Sivaguru, M., Hess, R. A., Nakamura, M. T. Deficiency in the omega-3 fatty acid pathway results in failure of acrosome biogenesis in mice. *Biology of reproduction* 2011; 85:721-32.

[79] Bel, S., Elkis, Y., Lerer-Goldstein, T., Nyska, A., Shpungin, S., Nir, U. Loss of TMF/ARA160 protein renders colonic mucus refractory to bacterial colonization and diminishes intestinal susceptibility to acute colitis. *The Journal of biological chemistry* 2012; 287:25631-9.

[80] Miller, V. J., Sharma, P., Kudlyk, T. A., Frost, L., Rofe, A. P., Watson, I. J., Duden, R., Lowe, M., Lupashin, V. V., Ungar, D. Molecular Insights into Vesicle Tethering at the Golgi by the Conserved Oligomeric Golgi (COG) Complex and the Golgin TATA Element Modulatory Factor (TMF). *J. Biol. Chem.* 2013; 288:4229-40.

[81] Lerer-Goldshtein, T., Bel, S., Shpungin, S., Pery, E., Motro, B., Goldstein, R. S., Bar-Sheshet, S. I., Breitbart, H., Nir, U. TMF/ARA160: A key regulator of sperm development. *Developmental biology* 2010; 348:12-21.

[82] Salcini, A. E., Confalonieri, S., Doria, M., Santolini, E., Tassi, E., Minenkova, O., Cesareni, G., Pelicci, P. G., DiFiore, P. P. Binding specificity and *in vivo* targets of the EH domain, a novel protein-protein interaction module. *Gene Dev.* 1997; 11:2239-49.

[83] Kang-Decker, N., Mantchev, G. T., Juneja, S. C., McNiven, M. A., van Deursen, J. M. Lack of acrosome formation in Hrb-deficient mice. *Science* 2001; 294:1531-3.

[84] Bennett, E. P., Hassan, H., Clausen, H. cDNA cloning and expression of a novel human UDP-N-acetyl-alpha-D-galactosamine - Polypeptide N-acetylgalactosaminyltransferase, GalNAc-T3. *J. Biol. Chem.* 1996; 271: 17006-12.

[85] Miyazaki, T., Mori, M., Yoshida, C. A., Ito, C., Yamatoya, K., Moriishi, T., Kawai, Y., Komori, H., Kawane, T., Izumi, S. et al. Galnt3 deficiency disrupts acrosome formation and leads to oligoasthenoteratozoospermia. *Histochemistry and cell biology* 2013; 139:339-54.

[86] Ramalho-Santos, J., Moreno, R. D. Targeting and fusion proteins during mammalian spermiogenesis. *Biol. Res.* 2001; 34:147-52.

[87] West, A. P., Willison, K. R. Brefeldin A and mannose 6-phosphate regulation of acrosomic related vesicular trafficking. *European journal of cell biology* 1996; 70:315-21.

[88] Li, Y. C., Hu, X. Q., Zhang, K. Y., Guo, H., Hu, Z. Y., Tao, S. X., Xiao, L. J., Wang, Q. Z., Han, C. S., Liu, Y. X. Afaf, a novel vesicle membrane protein, is related to acrosome formation in murine testis. *Febs Lett.* 2006; 580:4266-73.

[89] Berruti, G., Ripolone, M., Ceriani, M. USP8, a Regulator of Endosomal Sorting, Is Involved in Mouse Acrosome Biogenesis Through Interaction with the Spermatid ESCRT-0 Complex and Microtubules. *Biology of reproduction* 2010; 82:930-9.

[90] Qiao, Y., Yang, J. X., Zhang, X. D., Liu, Y., Zhang, J. C., Zong, S. D., Miao, S. Y., Wang, L. F., Koide, S. S. Characterization of rtSH3p13 gene encoding a development protein involved in vesicular traffic in spermiogenesis. *Cell Res.* 2004; 14:197-207.

[91] Li, S. C., Qiao, Y., Di, Q., Le, X. N., Zhang, L., Zhang, X. S., Zhang, C. Y., Cheng, J., Zong, S. D., Koide, S. S. et al. Interaction of SH3P13 and DYDC1 protein: a germ cell component that regulates acrosome biogenesis during spermiogenesis. *European journal of cell biology* 2009; 88:509-20.

[92] Schurmann, A., Axer, H., Scheepers, A., Doege, H., Joost, H. G. The glucose transport facilitator GLUT8 is predominantly associated with the acrosomal region of mature spermatozoa. *Cell and tissue research* 2002; 307:237-42.

[93] Augustin, R., Riley, J., Moley, K. H. GLUT8 contains a [DE]XXXL[LI] sorting motif and localizes to a late endosomal/lysosomal compartment. *Traffic* 2005; 6:1196-212.

[94] Hicke, L., Dunn, R. Regulation of membrane protein transport by ubiquitin and ubiquitin-binding proteins. *Annu. Rev. Cell Dev. Bi.* 2003; 19:141-72.

[95] Gnesutta, N., Ceriani, M., Innocenti, M., Mauri, I., Zippel, R., Sturani, E., Borgonovo, B., Berruti, G., Martegani, E. Cloning and characterization of mouse UBPy, a deubiquitinating enzyme that interacts with the Ras guanine nucleotide exchange factor CDC25(Mm)/ Ras-GRF1. *J. Biol. Chem.* 2001; 276:39448-54.

[96] Kato, M., Miyazawa, K., Kitamura, N. A deubiquitinating enzyme UBPY interacts with the Src homology 3 domain of Hrs-binding protein via a novel binding motif PX(V/I)(D/N)RXXKP. *J. Biol. Chem.* 2000; 275:37481-7.

[97] Quenneville, N. R., Chao, T. Y., McCaffery, J. M., Conibear, E. Domains within the GARP subunit Vps54 confer separate functions in complex assembly and early endosome recognition. *Molecular biology of the cell* 2006; 17:1859-70.

[98] Liewen, H., Meinhold-Heerlein, I., Oliveira, V., Schwarzenbacher, R., Luo, G. R., Wadle, A., Jung, M., Pfreundschuh, M., Stenner-Liewen, F. Characterization of the human GARP (Golgi associated retrograde protein) complex. *Experimental cell research* 2005; 306:24-34.

[99] Paiardi, C., Pasini, M. E., Gioria, M., Berruti, G. Failure of acrosome formation and globozoospermia in the wobbler mouse, a Vps54 spontaneous recessive mutant. *Spermatogenesis* 2011; 1:52-62.

[100] Tran, T. H. T., Zeng, Q., Hong, W. J. VAMP4 cycles from the cell surface to the trans-Golgi network via sorting and recycling endosomes. *Journal of cell science* 2007; 120:1028-41.

[101] Guo, X. J., Shen, J., Xia, Z. R., Zhang, R., Zhang, P., Zhao, C., Xing, J., Chen, L., Chen, W., Lin, M. et al. Proteomic Analysis of Proteins Involved in Spermiogenesis in Mouse. *J. Proteome Res.* 2010; 9:1246-56.

[102] Hamm-Alvarez, S. F., Sheetz, M. P. Microtubule-dependent vesicle transport: modulation of channel and transporter activity in liver and kidney. *Physiological reviews* 1998; 78:1109-29.

[103] Kraemer, J., Schmitz, F., Drenckhahn, D. Cytoplasmic dynein and dynactin as likely candidates for microtubule-dependent apical targeting of pancreatic zymogen granules. *European journal of cell biology* 1999; 78:265-77.

[104] Kamal, A., Goldstein, L. S. Connecting vesicle transport to the cytoskeleton. *Curr. Opin. Cell Biol.* 2000; 12:503-8.

[105] DePina, A. S., Langford, G. M. Vesicle transport: the role of actin filaments and myosin motors. *Microscopy research and technique* 1999; 47:93-106.

[106] Kierszenbaum, A. L., Rivkin, E., Tres, L. L. Cytoskeletal track selection during cargo transport in spermatids is relevant to male fertility. *Spermatogenesis* 2011; 1:221-30.

[107] Kierszenbaum, A. L., Rivkin, E., Tres, L. L. The actin-based motor myosin Va is a component of the acroplaxome, an acrosome-nuclear envelope junctional plate, and of manchette-associated vesicles. *Cytogenet. Genome Res.* 2003; 103:337-44.

[108] Kierszenbaum, A. L., Tres, L. L., Rivkin, E., Kang-Decker, N. L., van Deursen, J. M. A. The acroplaxome is the docking site of golgi-derived myosin Va/Rab27a/b-containing proacrosomal vesicles in wild-type and Hrb mutant mouse spermatids. *Biology of reproduction* 2004; 70:1400-10.

[109] Moreno, R. D., Palomino, J., Schatten, G. Assembly of spermatid acrosome depends on microtubule organization during mammalian spermiogenesis. *Developmental biology* 2006; 293:218-27.

[110] Huang, W. P., Ho, H. C. Role of microtubule-dependent membrane trafficking in acrosomal biogenesis. *Cell and tissue research* 2006; 323: 495-503.

[111] Yang, W. X., Sperry, A. O. C-terminal kinesin motor KIFC1 participates in acrosome biogenesis and vesicle transport. *Biology of reproduction* 2003; 69:1719-29.
[112] Goetz, S. C., Anderson, K. V. The primary cilium: a signalling centre during vertebrate development. *Nature reviews Genetics* 2010; 11:331-44.
[113] Kierszenbaum, A. L., Rivkin, E., Tres, L. L., Yoder, B. K., Haycraft, C. J., Bornens, M., Rios, R. M. GMAP210 and IFT88 are present in the spermatid golgi apparatus and participate in the development of the acrosome-acroplaxome complex, head-tail coupling apparatus and tail. *Developmental dynamics: an official publication of the American Association of Anatomists* 2011; 240:723-36.
[114] Lehman, J. M., Michaud, E. J., Schoeb, T. R., Aydin-Son, Y., Miller, M., Yoder, B. K. The Oak Ridge Polycystic Kidney mouse: modeling ciliopathies of mice and men. *Developmental dynamics: an official publication of the American Association of Anatomists* 2008; 237:1960-71.
[115] Schroer, T. A. Dynactin. *Annu. Rev. Cell Dev. Bi.* 2004; 20:759-79.
[116] Gillingham, A. K., Tong, A. H., Boone, C., Munro, S. The GTPase Arf1p and the ER to Golgi cargo receptor Erv14p cooperate to recruit the golgin Rud3p to the cis-Golgi. *The Journal of cell biology* 2004; 167:281-92.
[117] Rios, R. M., Tassin, A. M., Celati, C., Antony, C., Boissier, M. C., Homberg, J. C., Bornens, M. A peripheral protein associated with the cis-Golgi network redistributes in the intermediate compartment upon brefeldin A treatment. *The Journal of cell biology* 1994; 125:997-1013.
[118] Drin, G., Morello, V., Casella, J. F., Gounon, P., Antonny, B. Asymmetric tethering of flat and curved lipid membranes by a golgin. *Science* 2008; 320:670-3.
[119] Kramer, H., Phistry, M. Genetic analysis of hook, a gene required for endocytic trafficking in Drosophila. *Genetics* 1999; 151:675-84.
[120] Mendoza-Lujambio, I., Burfeind, P., Dixkens, C., Meinhardt, A., Hoyer-Fender, S., Engel, W., Neesen, J. The Hook1 gene is non-functional in the abnormal spermatozoon head shape (azh) mutant mouse. *Hum. Mol. Genet.* 2002; 11:1647-58.
[121] Berruti, G., Paiardi, C. USP8/UBPy-regulated sorting and the development of sperm acrosome: the recruitment of MET. *Reproduction* 2015; 149:633-44.

[122] Kierszenbaum, A. L., Rivkin, E., Tres, L. L. Acroplaxome, an F-actin-keratin-containing plate, anchors the acrosome to the nucleus during shaping of the spermatid head. *Molecular biology of the cell* 2003; 14: 4628-40.

[123] Fujihara, Y., Satouh, Y., Inoue, N., Isotani, A., Ikawa, M., Okabe, M. SPACA1-deficient male mice are infertile with abnormally shaped sperm heads reminiscent of globozoospermia. *Development* 2012; 139: 3583-9.

[124] Lin, Y. N., Roy, A., Yan, W., Burns, K. H., Matzuk, M. M. Loss of zona pellucida binding proteins in the acrosomal matrix disrupts acrosome biogenesis and sperm morphogenesis. *Molecular and cellular biology* 2007; 27:6794-805.

[125] Yu, Y., Vanhorne, J., Oko, R. The origin and assembly of a zona pellucida binding protein, IAM38, during spermiogenesis. *Microscopy research and technique* 2009; 72:558-65.

[126] Behnen, M., Murk, K., Kursula, P., Cappallo-Obermann, H., Rothkegel, M., Kierszenbaum, A. L., Kirchhoff, C. Testis-expressed profilins 3 and 4 show distinct functional characteristics and localize in the acroplaxome-manchette complex in spermatids. *Bmc Cell Biol.* 2009; 10.

[127] Obermann, H., Raabe, I., Balvers, M., Brunswig, B., Schulze, W., Kirchhoff, C. Novel testis-expressed profilin IV associated with acrosome biogenesis and spermatid elongation. *Mol. Hum. Reprod.* 2005;11:53-64.

[128] Rivkin, E., Kierszenbaum, A. L., Gil, M., Tres, L. L. Rnf19a, a Ubiquitin Protein Ligase, and Psmc3, a Component of the 26S Proteasome, Tether to the Acrosome Membranes and the Head-Tail Coupling Apparatus During Rat Spermatid Development. *Dev. Dynam.* 2009; 238:1851-61.

[129] Kierszenbaum, A. L., Rivkin, E., Talmor-Cohen, A., Shalgi, R., Tres, L. L. Expression of Full-Length and Truncated Fyn Tyrosine Kinase Transcripts and Encoded Proteins During Spermatogenesis and Localization During Acrosome Biogenesis and Fertilization. *Molecular reproduction and development* 2009; 76:832-43.

[130] Greer, P. Closing in on the biological functions of FPS/FES and FER. *Nat. Rev. Mol. Cell Bio.* 2002; 3:278-89.

[131] Kierszenbaum, A. L. Tyrosine protein kinases and spermatogenesis: Truncation matters. *Molecular reproduction and development* 2006; 73: 399-403.

[132] Kierszenbaum, A. L., Rivkin, E., Tres, L. L. Expression of Fer Testis (FerT) Tyrosine Kinase Transcript Variants and Distribution Sites of FerT During the Development of the Acrosome-Acroplaxome-Manchette Complex in Rat Spermatids. *Dev. Dynam.* 2008; 237:3882-91.

[133] Pierre, V., Martinez, G., Coutton, C., Delaroche, J., Yassine, S., Novella, C., Pernet-Gallay, K., Hennebicq, S., Ray, P. F., Arnoult, C. Absence of Dpy19l2, a new inner nuclear membrane protein, causes globozoospermia in mice by preventing the anchoring of the acrosome to the nucleus. *Development* 2012; 139:2955-65.

[134] Dittmer, T., Misteli, T. The lamin protein family. *Genome Biol.* 2011; 12.

[135] Shen, J., Chen, W., Shao, B. B., Qi, Y. J., Xia, Z. R., Wang, F. Q., Wang, L., Guo, X. J., Huang, X. Y., Sha, J. H. Lamin A/C proteins in the spermatid acroplaxome are essential in mouse spermiogenesis. *Reproduction* 2014; 148:479-87.

[136] Xu, X., Toselli, P. A., Russell, L. D., Seldin, D. C. Globozoospermia in mice lacking the casein kinase II alpha' catalytic subunit. *Nat. Genet.* 1999; 23:118-21.

[137] Kierszenbaum, A. L., Tres, L. L. The acrosome-acroplaxome-manchette complex and the shaping of the spermatid head. *Archives of histology and cytology* 2004; 67:271-84.

[138] Kierszenbaum, A. L., Rivkin, E., Tres, L. L. Molecular biology of sperm head shaping. *Society of Reproduction and Fertility supplement* 2007; 65:33-43.

[139] Morphogenesis of the acrosome during Upadhyay, R. D., Kumar, A. V., Ganeshan, M., Balasinor, N. H. Tubulobulbar complex: Cytoskeletal remodeling to release spermatozoa. *Reprod. Biol. Endocrin.* 2012; 10.

[140] Kopera, I. A., Bilinska, B., Cheng, C. Y., Mruk, D. D. Sertoli-germ cell junctions in the testis: a review of recent data. *Philosophical transactions of the Royal Society of London Series B, Biological sciences* 2010; 365:1593-605.

[141] Tanii, I., Yoshinaga, K., Toshimori, K. Morphogenesis of the acrosome during the final steps of rat spermiogenesis with special reference to tubulobulbar complexes. *Anat. Rec.* 1999; 256:195-201.

[142] Hartree, E. F. The acrosome-lysosome relationship. *Journal of reproduction and fertility* 1975; 44:125-6.

[143] Raposo, G., Marks, M. S., Cutler, D. F. Lysosome-related organelles: driving post-Golgi compartments into specialisation. *Curr. Opin. Cell Biol.* 2007; 19:394-401.

[144] Dell'Angelica, E. C., Mullins, C., Caplan, S., Bonifacino, J. S. Lysosome-related organelles. *Faseb Journal* 2000; 14:1265-78.

[145] Huizing, M., Helip-Wooley, A., Westbroek, W., Gunay-Aygun, M., Gahl, W. A. Disorders of lysosome-related organelle biogenesis: Clinical and molecular genetics. *Annu. Rev. Genom. Hum. G.* 2008; 9: 359-86.

[146] De Braekeleer, M., Nguyen, M. H., Morel, F., Perrin, A. Genetic aspects of monomorphic teratozoospermia: a review. *Journal of assisted reproduction and genetics* 2015; 32:615-23.

BIOGRAPHICAL SKETCH

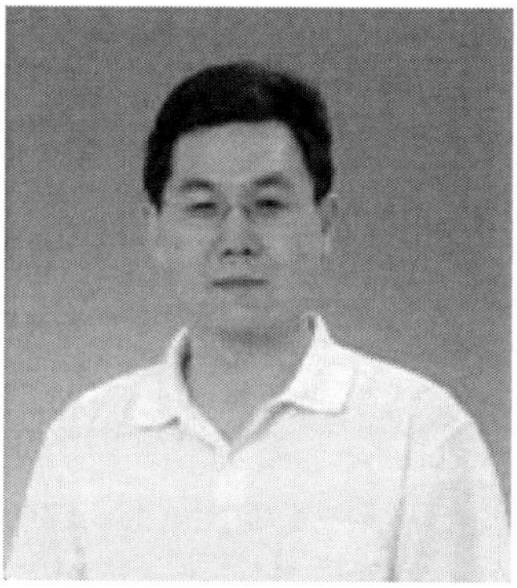

Wei Li got his Bachelor and PhD degree from Lanzhou University in 1998 and 2003, respectively. From 2003-2005, he worked on yeast molecular genetics for two years as a postdoctoral research fellow in the Department of Biological Sciences and Biotechnology, Tsinghua University. Then from 2005-2009, he worked on the mechanism of polyubiquitination as a postdoctoral visiting fellow in NIDDK/National Institutes of Health, US. In 2009 he joined the State Key Laboratory of Stem Cell and Reproductive Biology in the Institute of Zoology, CAS, as a principle investigator. His research focuses on the mechanisms of protein modification and their roles in reproduction and aging.

Publications Last 3 Years:

1. Zhang, P., He, Q., Chen, D., Liu, W., Wang, L., Zhang, C., Ma, D., Li, W., Liu, B., Liu, F. G protein-coupled receptor 183 facilitates endothelial-to-hematopoietic transition via Notch1 inhibition. *Cell Res.* 2015 Oct;25(10):1093-107.
2. Wang, Q., Liu, C., Tang, C., Guo, H., Liu, Y., Wang, L., Zhao, H., Shang, Y., Wen, Y., Lin, Y., Zhou, T., Zhou, Z., Dong, W., Hu, Z., Guo, X., Sha, J., Li, W*. Yeast model identifies ENTPD6 as a potential non-obstructive azoospermia pathogenic gene. *Sci. Rep.* 2015 Jul. 8;5:11762. doi: 10.1038/srep11762.
3. Song, Z. H., Yu, H. Y., Wang, P., Mao, G. K., Liu, W. X., Li, M. N., Wang, H. N., Shang, Y. L., Liu, C., Xu, Z. L., Sun, Q. Y., Li, W.*, Germ cell specific *Atg7* knockout results in primary ovarian insufficiency in female mice. *Cell Death Dis*. 2015 Jan. 15;6:e1589. doi: 10.1038/cddis. 2014.559.
4. Liu, W. X., Shang, Y. L., Li, W*. gp78 G2BR and CUE domains cooperatively elongate polyubiquitin chains from the distal end. *Sci. Rep.* 2014 Nov. 20;4:7138. doi: 10.1038/srep07138.
5. Wang, H. N., Wan, H. F., Li, X. X., Liu, W. X., Chen, Q., Wang, Y. Q., Yang, L., Duan, E. K., Tang, H. M., Zhang, X. J., Zhao, X. Y., Gao, F.*, Li, W*. Atg7 is required to acrosome biogenesis during mammalian spermatogenesis. *Cell Res.*, 2014 Jul;24(7):852-69.
6. Li, Y., Wu, H., Wu, W., Zhuo, W., Liu, W., Zhang, Y., Cheng, M., Chen, Y. G., Gao, N., Yu, H., Wang, L.*, Li, W.*, Yang, M*. Structural insights into the TRIM family of ubiquitin E3 ligases. *Cell Res*. 2014 Jun; 24(6):762-5.
7. Chen, M., Wang, X., Wang, Y., Zhang, L., Xu, B., Lv, L., Cui, X., Li, W.*, Gao, F*. Wt1 is involved in leydig cell steroid hormone biosynthesis by regulating paracrine factor expression in mice. *Biol. Reprod.* 2014 Apr. 3;90(4):71, 1-9.
8. Yan, L., Liu, W. X., Zhang, H. H., Liu, C., Shang, Y. L., Ye, Y. H., Zhang, X. D.*, Li, W.*, Ube2g2-gp78-mediated Herp polyubiquitination is involved in ER stress recovery. *J. Cell Sci.* 2014 Apr. 1;127: 1417-27.
9. Liu, W. X., Shang, Y. L., Zeng, Y., Liu, C., Li, Y. C., Zhai, L. H., Wang, P., Lou, J. Z., Xu, P., Ye, Y.*, Li, W*. Dimeric Ube2g2 simultaneously engages donor and acceptor ubiquitins to form Lys48-linked ubiquitin chains. *EMBO J.* 2014 Jan. 1;33(1):46-61.

10. Liu, Z., Ma, L., Wen, Z. S., Hu, Z., Wu, F. Q., Li, W., Liu, J., Zhou, G. B. Cancerous inhibitor of PP2A is targeted by natural compound celastrol for degradation in non-small-cell lung cancer. *Carcinogenesis*. 2014 Apr;35(4):905-14.
11. Qian, M. X., Pang, Y., Liu, C. H., Haratake, K., Du, B. Y., Ji, D. Y., Wang, G. F., Zhu, Q. Q., Song, W., Yu, Y., Zhang, X. X., Huang, H. T., Miao, S., Chen, L. B., Zhang, Z. H., Liang, Y. N., Liu, S., Cha, H., Yang, D., Zhai, Y., Komatsu, T., Tsuruta, F., Li, H., Cao, C., Li, W., Li, G. H., Cheng, Y., Chiba, T., Wang, L., Goldberg, A. L., Shen, Y., Qiu, X. B. Acetylation-mediated proteasomal degradation of core histones during DNA repair and spermatogenesis. *Cell.* 2013 May 23;153 (5): 1012-24.

In: Spermatogenesis
Editor: Gladys Robinson

ISBN: 978-1-63484-715-5

Chapter 2

REGULATORY ROLE OF NONCODING RNAS DURING SPERMATOGENESIS

Wenxian Zeng[1,*], Chuanying Pan[1,*] and Wan-Sheng Liu[2,†]

[1]College of Animal Science and Technology,
Northwest A&F University, Yangling, Shaanxi, P.R. China
[2]Department of Animal Science, Center for Reproductive Biology
and Health (CRBH), College of Agricultural Sciences,
The Pennsylvania State University, University Park, PA, US

ABSTRACT

Spermatogenesis is a continuous and organized process that occurs throughout the adult life of a male, by which spermatogonia proceed through mitosis, meiosis and complex cytological transformations resulting in the formation of spermatozoa. This process requires precise and highly ordered regulation of gene expression at both the transcriptional and posttranscriptional levels. Recent advances in genome-wide analyses of the mammalian transcriptome have revealed that in addition to mRNAs, several types of noncoding RNAs (ncRNAs), including microRNAs (miRNAs), endogenous small-interfering RNAs (endo-siRNAs), PIWI-interacting RNAs (piRNAs) and long noncoding RNAs (lncRNAs), are extensively transcribed during testis development

[*] These authors contributed equally to this work.
[†] Corresponding author: Telephone: 814 867 1673; Email: wul12@psu.edu.

and spermatogenesis. These ncRNAs are expressed in a cell-specific and step-specific manner to participate in the control of germ cell differentiation during spermatogenesis. In this review, we first briefly address the basics of spermatogenesis and the synthesis of ncRNAs, and then we discuss the recent progress in understanding of the functions of miRNAs, endo-siRNAs, piRNAs and lncRNAs in the regulation of spermatogenesis.

INTRODUCTION

Spermatogenesis occurs entirely within the seminiferous tubules in the testis throughout the adult life of a male. It is a highly complex process of molecular and cellular events in which spermatogonia mitotically divide, undergo meiosis and morphologic changes, then differentiate into motile spermatozoa (Schulz and Miura, 2002). Spermatogenesis starts with spermatogonial stem cells (SSCs), which are located in the basal compartment of seminiferous epithelium and are capable of self-renewal and differentiation, thereby giving rise to the entire spermatogenic lineage (de Rooij and Russell, 2000) (Figure 1). In rodents, spermatogonia are transformed from prospermatogonia shortly after birth and enter into mitotic proliferation. During the proliferation phase, spermatogonia are recognized as different subtypes, such as A1-A4 spermatogonia, intermediate spermatogonia, and B spermatogonia, among which SSCs are type A spermatogonia that process stem cell capacity (Phillips et al., 2010). Type B spermatogonia divide forming the primary spermatocytes, which proceed through meiosis I to produce secondary spermatocytes, and meiosis II to produce haploid round spermatids. The round spermatids then undergo a dramatic differentiation process termed spermiogenesis, which includes formation of the acrosome and flagellum, nuclear condensation, reorganization and compaction of the chromatin, cytoplasmic exclusion, and finally, giving rise to spermatozoa. Morphological criteria have been used to classify mouse spermiogenesis in 16 developmental steps (Oakberg, 1956). Based on cellular and nuclear shape, together with the stage of acrosomal and flagellar development, spermatids are divided into round (steps 5–8), elongating (steps 9–11), condensing (steps 12–14), and condensed (steps 14–16) spermatids (Cacciola et al., 2013; Oakberg, 1956). During the early steps, round spermatids are transcriptionally active, and the transcriptional activity in elongating spermatids decreases and then turns off (Paronetto and Sette, 2010). In this process, most of the histones in nucleosomes are replaced by transition proteins and subsequently by protamines (Marushige and Dixon, 1969) (Figure 1). The replacement is facilitated by incorporation of histone variants, posttranslational histone modifications, chromatin remodeling complexes, as well as transient DNA strand breaks (Rathke et al., 2014).

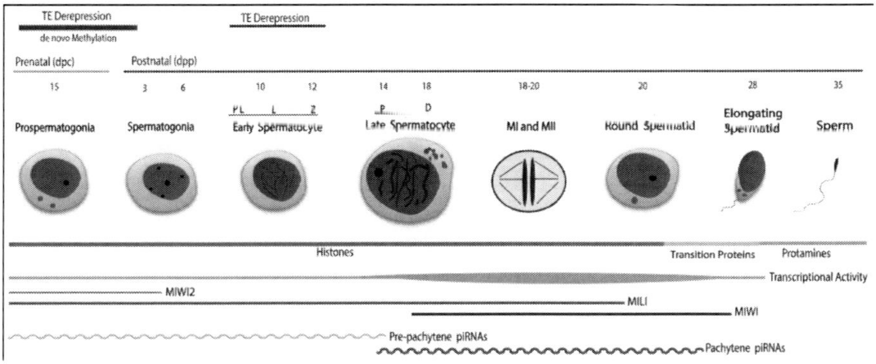

Figure 1. Male germ cell differentiation and the first wave of spermatogenesis in mouse. Primordial germ cells (PGCs) in prenatal testis transformed into prospermatogonia around 13.5 days post-coitum (dpc). After birth, germ cells begin differentiation by mitotic proliferation of spermatogonia, enter the meiotic pathway and become spermatocytes. Meiosis includes several phases (PL, preleptotene; L, leptotene; Z, zygotene; P, pachytene; D, diplotene), during which synaptonemal complex formation, crossing over and homologous recombination take place. Two subsequent divisions (MI and MII) at the end of the meiotic phase generate haploid round spermatids that undergo a dramatic differentiation programme (i.e., spermiogenesis). The approximate timing of the appearance of specific cell types during the first wave of spermatogenesis in juvenile mice is indicated as day postpartum (dpp). In elongating spermatids, chromatin is tightly compacted by replacing histones initially with transition proteins at 20-27 dpp and subsequently with protamines around 28 dpp. Gene expression is active during early spermatogenesis, particularly in late spermatocytes and round spermatids. Due to the chromatin packing, transcription ceases in elongating spermatids and mature sperm. The germ granules in prospermatogonia (pi-bodies and piR-bodies), late spermatocytes (intermitochondrial cement, IMC) and haploid spermatids (chromatoid body, CB) are shown in red. The formation of CB starts in late spermatocytes and is compacted to its characteristic form in early round spermatids. In elongating spermatids the CB is functionally transformed, and decreases in size and finally disappears. Pre-pachytene piRNAs are expressed together with Miwi2 and Mili in prenatal prospermatogonia. Their expression coincides with the nonproliferative phase of these cells (around 15 dpc – 3 dpp) during which they undergo a dramatic resetting of DNA methylation to generate novel gametic epigenetic marks by *de novo* methylation. The expression of transposable elements (TE) is derepressed during this time. There is a second transient derepression of transposons in early meiotic cells. In these cells, Mili is expressed together with pre-pachytene piRNAs. The massive induction of pachytene piRNA expression coincides with the appearance of the CB and expression of Miwi (Modified from Meikar et al., 2011).

Table 1. Characteristics of noncoding RNAs

Feature	miRNA	endo-siRNA	piRNA	lncRNA
Length	20-25 (nt)	~21 (nt)	24–32 (nt)	>200 (nt)
Number (in human)	~2588 (in miRBase)	Unknown	~6,000 clusters	~14,470
Processing protein AGO subfamily	Draosha/Dicer AGO	Dicer AGO	Zucchini PIWI	Unknown
Function in male germ cells	Self-renewal and differentiation of SSCs Promote apoptosis of SSCs Regulation of meiosis and spermatogenesis	Regulation of mRNA stability for spermatogenesis	Maintenance of genomic integrity Regulation germ cell proliferation, meiosis and spermiogenesis	Maintenance of SSC pool Spermatogonia differentiation
Mechanism in male germ cells	Translation repression RNA degradation	RNA cleavage	Silence of transposon Degradation of RNA Genomic imprinting Regulation of mRNA translation	Epigenetic regulation of gene expression Regulation of miRNA expression

This highly organized spermatogenesis requires timely coordinated gene expression that is regulated during transcription, posttranscriptional and epigenetic processes (Kimmins and Sassone-Corsi, 2005; Papaioannou and Nef, 2010). Previous studies have identified over a thousand protein coding genes that play a role in spermatogenesis (Hermo et al., 2010a-e; Waclawska and Kurpisz, 2012). However, molecular mechanisms involved in the regulation of transcription and translation of these genes have not been fully elucidated. Recent advances in genome-wide analyses of the mammalian transcriptome have revealed that several types of noncoding RNAs (ncRNAs), including microRNAs (miRNAs), endogenous small-interfering RNAs (endo-siRNAs), PIWI-interacting RNAs (piRNAs) and long noncoding RNAs (lncRNAs), are extensively transcribed during testis development and spermatogenesis (Table 1). These ncRNAs are expressed in a cell-specific and step-specific manner and are essential regulatory elements for mechanisms underlying germ cell differentiation during spermatogenesis (Figure 1).

Several recent review articles have summarized the role of ncRNAs in spermatogenesis and male fertility (de Mateo and Sassone-Corsi, 2014; Kotaja, 2014; He et al., 2009; Lee et al., 2009; Mukherjee et al., 2014; Wang and Xu, 2015; Yao et al., 2015; Zhang et al., 2014). In this chapter, we will focus on the most recent progress of ncRNAs, particularly lncRNAs, in the regulation of spermatogenesis.

MicroRNAs in Spermatogenesis

miRNAs Biogenesis

As of July 2015, a total of 1881 miRNA loci have been annotated in the human genome in the miRNA database (miRBase 21; http://www.mirbase.org). Similar number of miRNAs is expected to be identified in the mouse and other mammalian genomes (Table 1). The majority of these miRNA genes are intergenic or oriented antisense to neighboring genes and are likely transcribed as independent genes (Lagos-Quintana et al., 2001; Lau et al., 2001; Lee and Ambros, 2001; Lee et al., 2004). But in some cases a miRNA gene is transcribed together with its host gene, providing a means for coupled regulation of a miRNA and a protein-coding gene (Barik, 2008). Interestingly, about half of miRNA genes are organized in polycistronic clusters and are therefore coexpressed with a shared promoter (Truscott et al., 2016). miRNAs are transcribed by two RNase III proteins, Drosha and Dicer. The production of miRNAs in mammalian cells is regulated at multiple levels, including miRNA transcription, processing by Drosha and Dicer in the nucleus and cytoplasm respectively, and modification by RNA editing, RNA methylation, uridylation and adenylation (Ha and Kim, 2014). miRNAs are synthesized as hairpin loop precursors predominantly by RNA polymerase II. As illustrated in Figure 2, the initial transcripts are called the primary miRNAs (pri-miRNAs), which are variable in length ranging from several hundreds to thousands of nucleotides (nt) (Cai et al., 2004; Lee et al., 2004). The pri-miRNAs are methylated by RNA methyltransferase-like 3 (METTL3), marking them for recognition and processing by the DiGeorge syndrome critical region 8 (DGCR8) protein (Alarcon et al., 2015). The pri-miRNAs are then processed into ~70 nt long miRNA precursor (pre-miRNAs) by Drosha and its cofactor DGCR8 in the nucleus (Denli et al., 2004; Gregory et al., 2004; Han et al., 2004; Landthaler et al., 2004; Lee et al., 2003). The pre-miRNAs are then exported into the cytoplasm by exportin 5 (EXP5) in complex with Ran·GTP (Lund et al., 2004; Yi et al., 2003) and cleaved by Dicer into ~22 (19–25) base pair (bp) double-strands RNAs (dsRNAs) (Meister and Tuschl, 2004). These dsRNAs are loaded onto Argonaute (AGO) protein to assemble a miRNA-induced silencing complex (RISC), where one strand of the dsRNAs is retained as mature miRNA and the other strand is discarded during the RISC assembly (Lee et al., 2006) (Figure 2). RNA editing has been identified in ~6% of human miRNAs, which is a site-specific modification to yield RNA products different from those encoded by their DNA (of miRNA genes). This increases the diversity and space of miRNA action beyond that implicated from the genome alone (Blow et al., 2006). We encourage the readers who are interested in the molecular mechanism underlying miRNAs biogenesis to read the detailed review "Regulation of microRNA biogenesis" by Ha and Kim (2014).

Function of miRNAs in Spermatogenesis

miRNAs modulate the sequence-specific recognition of their target mRNAs by the RISC complex. The target mRNAs are either translationally repressed or degraded depending on sequence complementary (Martinez and Tuschl, 2004) (Figure 2). In addition, it has been recently shown that miRNAs regulate m6A modification in mRNAs via a sequence pairing mechanism (Chen et al., 2015). The methylated mRNAs, in turn, play pivotal physiological functions in regulating RNA metabolism and various biological processes, for instance, cell fate determination (Wang et al., 2014).

It is estimated that miRNAs target ~60% of protein-coding genes of humans and other mammals (Friedman et al., 2009; Lewis et al., 2005). One miRNA may target many genes, as many as 400 on average (Friedman et al., 2009). Conversely, multiple miRNAs may modulate the expression of a single gene (Sood et al., 2006). miRNAs are differentially expressed during development of testicular tissue (Buchold et al., 2010; Ro et al., 2007; Yan et al., 2007) and in the different types of male germ cells (Hayashi et al., 2008; Liu et al., 2015; Luo et al., 2015; Marcon et al., 2008; McIver et al., 2012a, b; Smorag et al., 2012; Tan et al., 2014; Wu et al., 2014a). Some miRNAs are commonly expressed among different types of germ cells, while other miRNAs are specifically expressed in certain cell types.

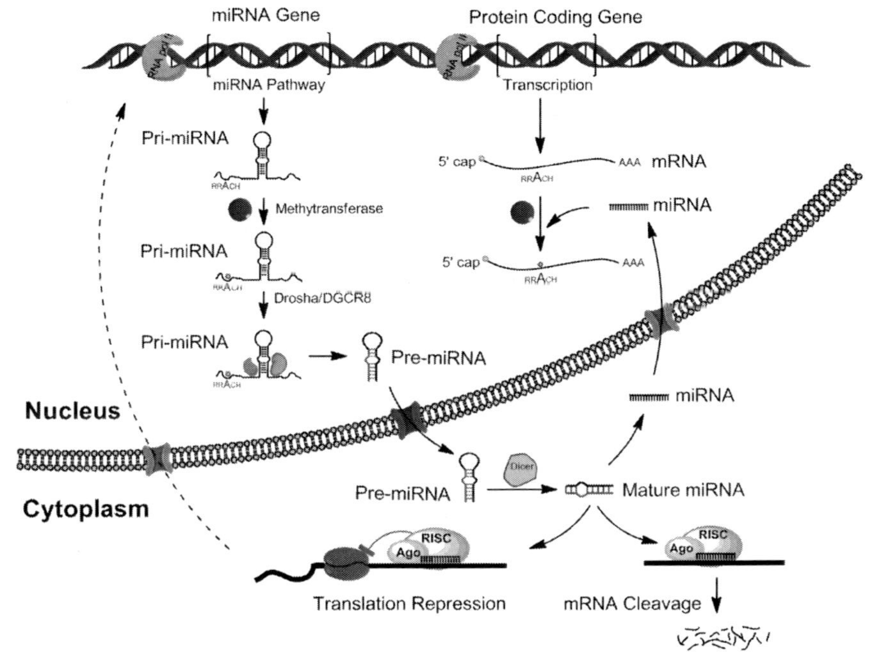

Figure 2. The biogenesis and function of miRNAs. miRNAs genes are transcribed into hairpin loop pri-miRNA by RNA pol Ⅱ or Ⅲ. Pri-miRNAs are methylated in the m6A position (red dot) of the sequence RRACH (R is a purine, and H is C, A, or U) by RNA methyltransferase (dark blue complex). The methylated pri-miRNAs are then recognized and processed by the microprocessor (Drosha-DGCR8) into pre-miRNAs that are ~70 nucleotides (nt) in length. Pre-miRNAs are transported to cytoplasm through the nuclear pore complex, where they are processed into ~22 (21-25) base pairs (bp) double-strands (ds) RNAs. These dsRNAs are then unwound, one of the strands is degraded and the other one is incorporated into Argonaute (AGO) protein to form RNA-induced silencing complex (RISC). Depending on the base pairing, target mRNAs are cleaved by RISC leading to mRNA cleavage or translational repression. The latter in turn regulates the expression of the corresponding miRNA genes in nucleus (dashed arrow). On the right side of the figure, mature miRNAs are imported into nucleus from cytoplasm via an unknown mechanism and regulate m6A methylation during mRNAs processing. The methylated mRNAs are involved in RNA metabolism and post-transcriptional gene expression regulation.

miRNAs contribute to maintenance of the pool of SSCs in the testis. It has been shown that miR-20, miR-21, miR-34c, miR-135a, miR-182, miR-183, miR-146a, miR-204, miR-544 were abundant in mammalian SSCs (He et al., 2013; Hua, 2015; Li et al., 2013; Moritoki et al., 2014). Interestingly, miR-20, miR-21, and miR-106a play an important role in regulating mouse SSC homeostasis (He et al., 2013; Niu et al., 2011). The miR-34c is also expressed in goat SSCs and promotes apoptosis of SSCs in a p53-dependent manner (Li et al., 2013). A recent study showed that miR-544 regulates self-renewal of goat SSC by targeting the promyelocytic leukemia zinc finger gene (*PLZF*) (Song et al., 2015). On the other hand, several miRNAs have been demonstrated to modulate differentiation of spermatogonia. miR-146 (Huszar and Payne, 2013), let 7 family miRNAs (Tong et al., 2011), miR-17-92 and miR-106b-25 clusters (Tong et al., 2012) have been found to be downregulated during retinoic acid (RA)-induced spermatogonial differentiation.

miRNAs play important roles in germ cells during meiosis and spermiogenesis. The miR-17-92 cluster protects meiotic germ cells from apoptosis by downregulation of translation of E2F transcription factor 1 (*E2f1*) (Novotny et al., 2007). MiR-18 is abundantly expressed in spermatocytes and plays a role in spermatogenesis by targeting heat shock factor 2 (*Hsf2*), which is a critical transcription factor in regulating male germ cell development in mice (Bjork et al., 2010). Moreover, miR-449 is significantly upregulated upon meiotic initiation during testis development and in adult mouse spermatogenesis. Intriguingly, the expression pattern of miR-449 resembles that of miR-34b/c during spermatogenesis (Bao et al., 2012; Wu et al., 2014b). Mutations at either the miR-449 locus or the miR-34 cluster do not cause a discernable phenotype on reproduction in male mice; however, inactivation of both the miR-449 and the miR-34 cluster results in infertility (Wu et al., 2014b). In addition to its roles in regulation of SSC fate, the miR-34c is highly expressed in mouse pachytene spermatocytes and spermatids. It regulates germ cell viability in mouse testis by targeting activating transcription factor 1 (*Atf1*) (Liang et al., 2012).

The timely expression of transition proteins (Tp) and protamines (Prm) is a prerequisite for compaction and condensation of chromatin during spermiogenesis (Meikar et al., 2013). MiR-469 represses Tp2 and Prm2 from translation by binding to target *Tp2* and *Prm2* mRNAs in pachytene spermatocytes and round spermatids (Dai et al., 2011). In contrast, miR-122a, which is highly expressed in late stage male germ cells, reduces the mRNA of *Tp2* by mRNA cleavage (Yu et al., 2005).

In summary, miRNAs are expressed in the testis and display germ cell-specific and developmentally regulated patterns of expression. miRNAs play indispensable roles in regulation of spermatogenesis, including the mitotic phase, meiotic phase, spermiogenesis, and final release of spermatozoa into the lumen of seminiferous tubules.

ENDOGENOUS SMALL-INTERFERING RNAS IN SPERMATOGENESIS

Endo-siRNAs Biogenesis

Unlike miRNAs, endo-siRNAs do not need the microprocessor complex (Drosha-DGCR8) for their biogenesis because they are processed from precursors of long double-stranded RNAs (dsRNA) that can be either sense or antisense RNA pairs or long hairpins (Krol et al., 2010; Suh et al., 2011) (Table 1). By investigation of *Drosha* or *Dicer* conditional knockout (cKO) mouse lines, Wu et al. demonstrated that the biosynthesis of mouse testicular endo-siRNAs requires Dicer activity, but is independent of Drosha (Wu et al., 2012). In Drosophila, a class of hairpin RNAs (hpRNAs) has been recently found to become an endo-siRNA class, which are predominantly expressed in testes (Wen et al., 2015).

Function of Endo-siRNAs in Spermatogenesis

Endo-siRNAs were initially reported in model organisms, such as Drosophila (Czech et al., 2008) and mouse (Garcia-Lopez et al., 2014, 2015; Song et al., 2011; Tam et al., 2008). In mice, embryonic stem cells (ESCs) express the most abundant endo-siRNAs, followed by SSCs, with the lowest levels in developing germ cells (Tan et al., 2014). Profiling of the small ncRNAs (sncRNAs) in primordial germ cells (PGCs), oocytes and zygotes indicates that both miRNAs and small nucleolar RNAs (snoRNAs) are abundantly expressed in PGCs, but transiently replaced by piRNAs in spermatozoa and endo-siRNAs in oocytes and zygotes (Garcia-Lopez et al., 2015).

In mice and other mammals, germ cell-specific inactivation of *Dicer* led to complete male infertility due to alterations in meiotic progression, increased spermatocyte apoptosis and defects in the maturation of spermatozoa (Zimmermann et al., 2014). *Drosha* KO mice with a defective miRNA pathway but intact endo-siRNA pathways displayed more severe spermatogenic disruptions than *Dicer* cKO mice, similar to results obtained with the *Dgcr8* KO mice. These studies reveal a role of endo-siRNAs in the progression of mammalian spermatogenesis and male fertility (Wu et al., 2012; Zimmermann et al., 2014).

It was proposed earlier that the presence and function of endo-siRNAs were restricted to germ cells, but recent studies have identified endo-siRNAs in different types of somatic cells, opening a new dimension for studying their regulatory roles (Carlile et al., 2009; Mirkovic-Hosle et al., 2014; Tam et al., 2008; Zhou et al., 2009). Further study is needed to elucidate the functions of endo-siRNA in spermatogenesis.

PIWI-Interacting RNAs in Spermatogenesis

piRNA and PIWI Machinery

piRNAs are a large class of small ncRNAs that are 24-32 nt in length and form RNA-protein complexes through interactions with PIWI proteins (Aravin et al., 2006, 2008; Girard et al., 2006; Grivna et al., 2006a; Lin, 2007), and are thus termed PIWI-interacting RNAs. PIWI proteins are a subfamily of the AGO protein family, and are predominantly expressed in mammalian male testes, whereas AGO proteins are ubiquitously expressed. The PIWI proteins are highly conserved across evolutionary lineages. Three Piwi proteins (Miwi, Miwi2, and Mili) are temporally and spatially expressed in mice during spermatogenesis. Miwi2 is expressed in prospermatogonia from 15.5 days postcoitum (dpc) to 3 days postpartum (dpp) (Aravin et al., 2008). Mili is expressed in prospermatogonia, spermatogonia, spermatocytes and round spermatids from 12.5 dpc to 20 dpp (Deng and Lin, 2002). While Miwi is expressed in the spermatocytes and the spermatids from 15 to 28 dpp (Deng and Lin, 2002) (Figure 1).

Genetic mutation of the *Piwi* gene affects the development of the male germline. Deficiency in *Mili* or *Miwi2* results in the activation of long interspersed nuclear elements (LINEs) and long terminal repeats (LTRs) retrotransposons including L1 and intracisternal A-particle (IAP) elements, and arrest of SSCs. Inactivation of Miwi leads to dysregulation of L1 transposons and spermiogenic arrest at the early spermatid stage (Reuter et al., 2011). Interestingly, unlike in mice, four PIWI proteins are expressed in human and marmoset testes, including PIWIL1/HIWI, PIWIL2/HILI, PIWIL3, and PIWIL4/HIWI2 (Hirano et al., 2014; Sasaki et al., 2003). However, the function of these proteins in primates is not fully understood.

The murine Piwi proteins and piRNAs are expressed in a developmental stage-specific manner (Figure 1). The proper clearance of these Piwi proteins and piRNAs is probably essential for male germ cell development and spermatogenesis. Recently, it has been found that piRNAs trigger Miwi ubiquitination by a multisubunit E3 ubiquitin ligase, APC/C (the anaphase promoting complex/cyclosome), at a later stage of spermatogenesis, thereby resulting in the degradation of Miwi via the ubiquitin-26S proteasome (Ub/26S) pathway. Importantly, such piRNA-triggered clearance of Miwi proteins that leads to the elimination of piRNAs themselves, suggests a feed-forward mechanism for coordinated removal of the Miwi/piRNA machinery after it accomplishes its function for spermatogenesis (Zhao et al., 2013). However, the mechanism by which Mili and Miwi2 proteins are degraded during spermatogenesis remains mysterious.

To date, a large number of piRNA-related sequences have been identified in mouse (Watanabe et al., 2015), human (Ha et al., 2014), and marmoset (Hirano et al., 2014) testes through RNA-seq technology. piRNAs are often present in clusters from few to hundreds of kilobase pairs (kb) in length, which are distributed throughout the genome (Aravin et al., 2007). piRNAs are featured with preference for a uridine at the 5′ end and the Hen1-mediated 2′-O-methylation at the 3′ end (Aravin et al., 2007; Siomi et al., 2011). Based on their expression at specific developmental stages during male germ cell development, piRNAs are grouped into two classes, prepachytene piRNAs and pachytene piRNAs. The chronological and overlapping expression patterns of Piwi proteins and piRNAs and their interactions during spermatogenesis are presented in Figure 1.

Prepachytene piRNAs

Prepachytene piRNAs include fetal and postnatal prepachytene piRNAs. Fetal prepachytene piRNAs are expressed in prospermatogonia and are associated with the Mili and Miwi2 proteins. Mili binds predominantly to piRNAs that are sense to transposable elements (TEs), while Miwi2 binds preferentially to piRNAs that are antisense to TEs (Aravin et al., 2008) (Figure 1). About half of fetal prepachytene piRNAs are derived from TEs. A small percentage (3%) of fetal prepachytene piRNAs are derived from the exons of protein-coding genes (Aravin et al., 2008).

Postnatal prepachytene piRNAs are associated only with Mili, which is the sole Piwi protein present at this stage. Similar to the fetal stage, approximately 50% of postnatal prepachytene piRNAs are derived from TEs. However, the profile of the TEs from which postnatal prepachytene piRNAs originate is different from that of TEs from which the fetal prepachytene piRNAs are derived. Compared to fetal prepachytene piRNAs, a greater percentage (20%) of postnatal prepachytene piRNAs are also derived from the exons of protein-coding genes (Aravin et al., 2008).

Pachytene piRNAs

The vast majority (95%) of the known piRNAs are pachytene piRNAs (the remaining 5% are prepachytene piRNAs) (Aravin et al., 2006, 2007; Gan et al., 2011; Girard et al., 2006; Grivna et al., 2006a). Pachytene piRNAs are differentially expressed in pachytene spermatocytes and round spermatids. They are associated with the Mili and Miwi proteins. Unlike prepachytene piRNAs, the majority (80%) of the pachytene piRNAs are derived from the piRNA clusters, which are nonrepetitive, intergenic DNA regions (Gan et al., 2011; Girard et al., 2006). These piRNAs have no known targets and are hypothesized to be the degradation products of larger ncRNAs that are selectively targeted for processing by the piRNA pathway (Vourekas et al., 2012). The remaining (~20%) pachytene piRNAs are derived from TEs (Aravin et al., 2006; Girard et al., 2006). Pachytene piRNA clusters are larger, on average, than prepachytene piRNA clusters. In addition, these two clusters usually do not overlap in the genome (Aravin et al., 2007).

piRNA Biogenesis

piRNAs are processed from the single-stranded RNA precursors that are mainly transcribed from two genomic sources, i.e., piRNA clusters and active transposons (TEs) (see above). Their biogenesis is Dicer-independent, thus it is distinct from that of miRNAs and endo-siRNAs (Gunawardane et al., 2007; Houwing et al., 2007; Saito et al., 2007; Vagin et al., 2006) (Table 1). After maturation, piRNAs associate with Piwi proteins to form piRNA-induced silencing complexes (piRISCs) and then direct piRISCs to target transcripts by means of RNA–RNA base-pairing. It is not fully understood how piRNAs are generated. Two distinct models have been proposed to date, i.e., the primary processing pathway and the ‘Ping-Pong cycle’ pathway (Fu and Wang, 2014; Guzzardo et al., 2013; Yadav and Kotaja, 2014).

Both the primary processing and the Ping-Pong cycle pathway are observed during fetal prepachytene piRNA biogenesis in mice, wherein primary piRNAs are loaded onto Mili, while the secondary piRNAs are loaded onto both Mili and Miwi2 (Aravin et al., 2008; De Fazio et al., 2011). However, piRNA biogenesis during adult spermatogenesis in mice is independent of the Ping-Pong mechanism (Beyret et al., 2012). While Miwi2 is involved in the linear generation of secondary piRNAs, Mili forms an intraamplification loop with itself to amplify piRNAs (De Fazio et al., 2011). Because Mili predominantly associates with fetal prepachytene piRNAs that are sense to TEs, it is believed that transcripts of TEs are fed into the piRNA pathway to generate the initial pool of primary piRNAs. Secondary piRNAs are antisense to TEs and guide Miwi2 to silence TEs in the nucleus. This mechanism allows germ cells to establish an adaptive defense against endogenous TEs through the piRNA pathway.

piRNA Function in Spermatogenesis

Silence of Transposons and Maintenance of Genome Integrity

piRNAs are involved in development, epigenetic regulation and transposon repression in mammalian male germ cells (Bao and Yan, 2012; Chuma et al., 2006). TEs and their evolutionary remnants are mobile DNA segments that may result in harmful insertional mutagenesis and/or genomic rearrangements when aberrantly expressed. If these mutations remain uncorrected, germ cells may enter apoptosis, resulting in sterility, or erroneous genome codes may appear in the next generation. Fortunately, expression of TEs is silenced in mammalian germ cells during transcription by DNA methylation on transposons, and posttranscriptional gene silencing occurs by cleavage of transposon transcripts (Aravin et al., 2008; Castaneda et al., 2014; Kuramochi-Miyagawa et al., 2008; Saxe et al., 2013; Siomi et al., 2011; Watanabe et al., 2011a). In this silencing pathway, primary piRNAs loaded to Piwi (Miwi2 and/or Mili) proteins recognize complementary target RNAs that are cleaved to generate secondary piRNAs that, in turn, continue the cycle to amplify the piRNA response, therefore silencing TEs and maintaining genomic integrity in prospermatogonia. It was found that silencing and *de novo* DNA methylation of L1 and IAP elements were decreased in male germ lines that were defective for the activity of the *Mili* or *Miwi2* gene (Aravin et al., 2007, 2008; Kuramochi-Miyagawa et al., 2008).

The connection between regulation of transposons by piRISCs and the defects in gametogenesis has not been established. It was proposed that activation of transposons in *Piwi* mutants might lead to the generation of dsDNA breaks that could cause a sterile phenotype (Klattenhoff et al., 2007).

In a case of spermiogenic arrest, loss of the piRNA biogenesis factor Maelstrom (Mael) in mouse was considered to be the causative reason (Castaneda et al., 2014). It is believed that tissue-specific and developmental stage–specific expression of Piwi and piRNAs may play major roles in maintaining the integrity of the genome and fertility of the species.

In addition to prepachytene piRNAs, pachytene piRNAs are also involved in silencing TEs. Loss of piRNAs results in derepression of transposable elements in adult meiotic and haploid germ cells, and ultimately male sterility characterized by a germ cell arrest at the steps 9–11 during spermatid elongation (Lim et al., 2015; Zheng and Wang, 2012). *Miwi*-KO mice display an increased level of LINE1 transcripts with high complementarity to pachytene piRNAs (Reuter et al., 2011). The increase in LINE1 in the absence of pachytene piRNAs is 10-fold less than that in the absence of prepachytene piRNA, suggesting that transposon silencing may be a minor role for pachytene piRNAs (Zheng and Wang, 2012; Zheng et al., 2010).

It has been shown that, in addition to DNA methylation, piRNAs epigenetically regulate TEs through histone methylation. In the nucleus, the piRISCs direct methylation of histone 3 lysine 9 (H3K9me3) on chromatin at target transposon loci to induce the formation of heterochromatin, thus transcriptionally silencing transposons (Bourc'his and Bestor, 2004; Di Giacomo et al., 2013; Hata et al., 2002; Morris et al., 2004; Song et al., 2004). Methyltransferases set domain bifurcated 1 (Setdb1), Su(var)3–9 and the heterochromatin protein 1α (Hp1a) are involved in the establishment of H3K9me3 on the silenced transposon loci (Ma et al., 2009; Shoji et al., 2009; Soper et al., 2008; Zheng et al., 2010). However, the mechanisms underlying the involvement of piRNAs in histone methylation is still not fully understood.

Degradation of RNAs

piRNAs act as siRNAs to degrade specific mRNAs in the mouse testis and the proper turnover of certain key piRNA targets is essential for sperm formation (Goh et al., 2015; Zhang et al., 2015). piRNAs also act as guide molecules to identify target RNAs and negatively regulate protein-coding mRNAs and L1 retrotransposons as well as lncRNAs in late spermatocytes (Goh et al., 2015). Interestingly, retrotransposons autoregulate the turnover of their own RNAs in the mouse testis using the same piRNAs pathway (Watanabe et al., 2015). Pachytene piRNAs bound to Miwi are responsible for eliminating the expression of bulk mRNAs in spermatids. The Miwi-piRISC forms a complex with a deadenylase, chromatin assembly factor 1 (Caf1), which promotes deadenylation and decay of a large population of mRNAs in elongating spermatids (Gou et al., 2014; Watanabe et al., 2015).

Genomic Imprinting

The imprinted genes are controlled by DNA methylation in the differentially methylated regions (DMRs) (Schaefer et al., 2007). During murine development, the DMRs are demethylated (erasure of imprint mark) in PGCs at 10.5 to 12.5 dpc and *de novo* methylated (reestablishment of imprinting) in prospermatogonia at 12.5 to 18.5 dpc (Schaefer et al., 2007). Therefore, spermatogonia maintain methylation patterns for the large and variable number of mitotic divisions that precede entry into meiosis. The imprinted Ras protein-specific guanine nucleotide-releasing factor 1 (*Rasgrf1)* locus, located in mouse chromosome 9, is methylated on the paternal allele within a differentially methylated domain 30 kp 5' of the promoter. Interestingly, a ncRNA transcribed from a retrotransposon-containing region, spanning the DMR of *Rasgrf1,* was targeted by piRNAs that were derived from transposons coded in chromosome 7. The piRNAs and the corresponding target RNA direct the sequence-specific methylation of *Rasgrf1* (Watanabe et al. 2011b). However, the molecular mechanism of this process remains unknown. It is likely that piRISCs may recruit DNA methyltransferase Dnmt3l to the DMR region of *Rasgrf1* gene (Watanabe et al. 2011b).

Regulation of mRNA Translation

It is unclear how piRNAs are involved in the regulation of translation. In mice, piRNAs and Miwi are associated with mRNAs in polysomes and ribonucleoprotein (RNP) fractions (Grivna et al., 2006a, b). Several members in the family of eukaryotic translation initiation factor (Eif), including Eif3A, Eif4E, and Eif4G, interact with the Piwi protein family (Grivna et al., 2006b). Miwi binds to Eif4E, while Mili binds to Eif3A. They interact with the Eif4G containing mRNA 5'cap-binding complex (Unhavaithaya et al., 2009).

Proteins Associated with PIWI/piRNA Machinery

In addition to Piwi, the piRNAs pathway is made up of other Piwi-associated proteins (Wasik et al., 2015). Discovery of these proteins has provided significant mechanistic insights into the Piwi/piRNA machinery. Several proteins from the tudor domain-containing protein (Tdrd) family have been found to be associated with Piwi and are required for spermatogenesis.

These Tdrds are believed to function as scaffolds for interaction of various proteins to form germ line granules (Chen et al., 2009). Several classes of germline granules have been observed in different types of germ cells (Figure 1). The chromatoid body (CB) is the most well studied granule to date. The CB is first visible in the cytoplasm of spermatocytes at mid-to-late meiotic stage and persistently develops in round spermatids (Chuma et al., 2009; Eddy, 1975). It moves toward the base of the flagellum and is finally discarded along with the cytoplasm in residual bodies. Many RNA-binding proteins that are involved in different RNA regulation pathways are localized in the CB (Meikar et al., 2011). Moreover, the CB largely accumulates both Miwi and piRNAs in round spermatids. Therefore, the CB may serve as a center for Miwi and piRNA function. In addition, the intermitochondrial cement (IMC), located between mitochondria, is present in prospermatogonia, spermatogonia, and mid-late pachytene spermatocytes (Figure 1). Many components of the piRNA pathway, including Mili, Moloney leukemia virus 10-like 1 (Mov10l1), ankyrin repeat, SAM and basic leucine zipper domain containing 1 (Asz1, also known as Gasz), DEAD (Asp-Glu-Ala-Asp) box polypeptide 4 (Ddx4), Tdrd1, Tdrkh, Miwi and Mael, are localized in the IMC (Aravin et al., 2009; Chuma et al., 2006).

Taking together, piRNAs are preferentially expressed in different types of male germ cells and play essential roles in regulation of spermatogenesis. However, a lot of outstanding questions remain to be addressed. First, the mechanisms underlying piRNAs biogenesis remains unclear. Secondly, piRNAs are massively accumulated in pachytene spermatocytes and degraded in elongated spermatids. The functions of these pachytene piRNAs and the mechanisms underlying degradation of mRNA and piRNAs during spermiogenesis are vague.

LONG NONCODING RNAS IN SPERMATOGENESIS

Classification of lncRNAs

lncRNAs are nonprotein-coding transcripts longer than 200 nt (Wapinski and Chang, 2011; Rinn and Chang, 2012). This somewhat arbitrary limit distinguishes lncRNAs from miRNAs, endo-siRNAs, piRNAs and other short RNAs. Unlike other sncRNAs, such as miRNAs that exhibit strong conservation across species, lncRNAs are usually species-specific and less conserved (Kutter et al., 2012; Pauli et al., 2012). A large number of lncRNA genes are present in the human genome. According to the human GENCODE (v20) project, there are at least 14,470 annotated, independent lncRNA genes (Coffey et al., 2011; Harrow et al., 2012). However, the vast majority of the lncRNA genes have not been characterized, only a very small number (287) of them have been analyzed and collected in the lncRNA database (http://www.lncrnadb.org/) (Quek et al., 2015) (Table 1).

lncRNAs can be classified into two classes, circular lncRNAs and linear lncRNAs, based on the transcription in genomic localization. Circular lncRNAs are generated either by head-to-tail circularization from exons with covalent joined ends (circRNAs) (Hansen et al., 2013; Jeck et al., 2013; Memczak et al., 2013; Salzman et al., 2012) or derived from the lariat introns (ciRNAs) (Zhang et al., 2013). circRNAs were first found in the 1970s in several eukaryotic RNA viruses (Hsu and Coca-Prados, 1979; Kolakofsky, 1976). Subsequently several other circRNAs produced from eukaryotic genomes were identified. For instance, *Sry* (sex-determining region Y) is flanked by long inverted repeats over 15.5 kb in length, and is highly expressed in murine testes. A circRNA is generated from the Sry-related repeat region that contains 16 miR-138 binding sites (Capel et al., 1993; Hansen et al., 2013). To date, thousands of circRNAs have been identified across species (including C. elegans, yeast, mice and human) via the application of next generation sequencing technology (Danan et al., 2012; Jeck et al., 2013; Memczak et al., 2013; Qin et al., 2015; Salzman et al., 2012; Zhang et al., 2013). Compared to the circRNAs, very limited information is available about the intron lariats-derived ciRNAs. Zhang et al. identified a few hundreds of ciRNAs in H9 and Hela cells by RNA-seq. These ciRNAs are short-lived intermediates transcripts during RNA splicing (Zhang et al., 2013).

The linear RNAs include small nucleolar lncRNAs (sno-lncRNAs), enhancer RNAs (eRNAs), natural antisense transcripts (NATs) and large intergenic ncRNAs (lincRNAs). Introns containing two small nucleolar RNAs (snoRNAs) are processed from their ends by the sno-ribonucleoprotein (snoRNP) machinery. These transcribed intronic RNA sequences between the two snoRNAs are not cleared during RNA splicing, thus resulting in generation of lncRNAs with snoRNA ends (sno-lncRNAs) (Yin et al., 2012). These sno-lncRNAs are capped with snoRNAs at both ends, thus lack both 5′ cap structures and 3′ poly(A) tails. In contrast, eRNAs are transcribed bidirectionally from enhancer regions, usually < 2 kb in length without poly(A) tails (De Santa et al., 2010; Kim et al., 2010). The mechanism of eRNAs processing is still a mystery. As the name indicated, lincRNAs are transcribed from intergenic regions and are variable in length (Cabili et al.,

2011; Derrien et al., 2012; Guttman et al., 2009). NATs are RNA molecules that are transcribed from the opposite DNA strand of the gene and overlap in part with the sense RNA. The regulatory roles of NATs and lincRNAs are broad and fundamental, involving in nearly every level of gene regulation from pretranscriptional, transcriptional to posttranscriptional by DNA-RNA, RNA-RNA or protein-RNA interactions (Faghihi and Wahlestedt, 2009; Rinn and Chang, 2012; Ulitsky and Bartel, 2013; Villegas and Zaphiropoulos, 2015).

Mechanistic Models of lncRNAs

The potential function of the characterized lncRNAs reported in lncRNAdb v2.0 includes sequence conservation, specific and regulated gene expression, epigenetics regulation, alternate splicing and differential stability (Cao, 2014; Luk et al., 2014; van Bakel et al., 2010). The mechanisms by which lncRNAs function in cells are still unclear and at least five different models have been proposed to date: precursor, recruiter, activator, competitor and miRNA regulator (Luk et al., 2014).

For the model of precursor, lncRNA HongrES2 is confirmed to be the precursor of a small RNA, termed mil-HongrES2. HongrES2 is cleaved into mil-HongrES2 by combining with RNase (Cai and Cullen, 2007; Ni et al., 2011). HongrES2 affects the maturation and capacitation of rat spermatozoa by downregulating the expression of protein carboxylesterase 7 (Ces7) in epididymis through its derived small RNA (Cai and Cullen, 2007; Ni et al., 2011). lncRNA Evf2 (also known as Dlx6os1, distal-less homeobox 6, opposite strand 1) recruits methyl CpG binding protein 2 (Mecp2), leading to DNA methylation, which further causes gene silencing (Berghoff et al., 2013). The lncRNA HOTAIR acts as an activator to bind the polycomb repressive complex 2 (Prc2) and lysine (K)-specific demethylase 1A (Lsd1) complex to regulate chromatin states and specifying the pattern of histone modifications on target genes (Marchese and Huarte, 2014). Furthermore, lncRNAs compete with transcription factors for DNA binding sites (Hung et al., 2011; Ng et al., 2013). Some lncRNAs complementarily bind to DNA molecules and hinder protein binding to specific antisense mRNA (Kraus et al., 2013). lncRNAs can also inhibit the miRNA-induced mRNA degradation and translation by competing for binding sites with miRNAs as well (Zhang et al., 2010).

lncRNAs are also regarded as a part of the miRNA interaction network via lncRNAs-miRNA interactions (Jalali et al., 2013). It is reported that lncRNA NLC1-C modulated miR-320a and miR-383 expression at the transcriptional level by binding to RNA-binding proteins to regulate human spermatogenesis (Lu et al., 2015).

lncRNA Profiling in Testis and Male Germ Cells

A total of 8265 lncRNAs were detected and 3025 were differentially expressed in a microarray analysis during the mouse postnatal testis development (Sun et al., 2013; Sun and Wu, 2015). It is estimated that ~30% of the genome is differentially expressed during the mouse testis development. Gene expression changes dramatically in the first few days after birth (0–6 dpp), at the beginning of meiosis (12–14 dpp), and along with the appearance of haploid gametes (20 dpp) (Shima et al. 2004). Recently, a time course study of the testis gene expression at 7, 14, 17, 21 and 28 dpp using RNA-seq identified 947 upregulated lncRNAs during the first wave of spermatogenesis in mice. These lncRNAs appeare to be highly specific to different time points during the germ cell development (Laiho et al., 2013). Another recent microarray-based study by Bao et al. compared the lncRNAs profiles at six time points (12.5 and 15.5 dpc; 7, 14, 21 dpp and adult). They identified thousands of lncRNAs that are up- or downregulated at these six critical time points during male germ cell development. In addition, most of these lncRNAs are associated with clusters of protein-coding genes that are usually located close to the lncRNAs in the genome. The expression level of these protein-coding genes are somehow related to that of the lncRNAs (Bao et al., 2013).

In addition, Liang et al. reported that a larger number of lncRNAs (3639) are specifically expressed type A spermatogonia, while a much smaller number of lncRNAs are expressed in pachytene spermatocytes (98) and round spermatids (166) in mice (Liang et al., 2014). In addition, lncRNAs were found to be accumulated during meiotic and spermiogenic stages in rats (Chalmel et al., 2014). These unique expression patterns of lncRNAs in different types of male germ cells signify their significance in spermatogenesis.

Functional lncRNAs in Spermatogenesis

Although thousands of potential lncRNAs have been identified in testes and male germ cells, only a few have been functionally annotated and characterized.

Meiotic Recombination Hot Spot Locus (Mrhl)

Mrhl RNA is a 2.4-kb mono-exonic lncRNA located in the nucleus. Downregulation of *Mrhl* RNA results in the cytoplasmic translocation of tyrosine-phosphorylated p68, probably via inhibiting the Wnt signaling pathway (Arun et al., 2012).

HongrES2

This 1.6-kb chimeric transcript, expressed specifically in the cauda region of the epididymis, is the precursor for a miRNA-like small RNA, mil-HongrES2 (Ni et al., 2011) as discussed earlier in this chapter. mil-HongrES2 suppresses the expression of the rodent Ces7 and inhibits its cholesterol esterase activity. Overexpression of mil-HongrES2 leads to retarded sperm capacitation, suggesting that lncRNA is a gatekeeper for sperm maturation in rat epididymis (Ni et al., 2011).

Testis-Specific X-Linked (Tsx)

Tsx was thought to be a protein-coding gene, but it is actually a lncRNA (Anguera et al., 2011). *Tsx* is specifically expressed in pachytene spermatocytes, while not in spermatogonia or round spermatids. *Tsx*-KO mice showed an abnormally high proportion of pachytene spermatocytes that had undergone apoptosis, suggesting that its role is critical for progression of meiosis (Anguera et al., 2011).

Dmrt1-Related Gene (Dmr)

The doublesex and mab-3 related transcription factor 1 (Dmrt1) protein, an essential transcription factor, promotes spermatogonial development by upregulating spermatogenesis and oogenesis-specific basic helix-loop-helix 1 (*Sohlh1*) and prevents premature meiosis by repressing stimulated by retinoic acid gene 8 (*Stra8*) (Agbor et al., 2013; Ottolenghi et al., 2000). The transcript from *Dmr* is a lncRNA, which is able to form a transsplicing RNA. The latter disrupts the coding region of *Dmrt1* and replaces the 3′-UTR of *Dmrt1*, leading to downregulation of the Dmrt1 protein (Zhang et al., 2010).

Spermatogonial-Specific lncRNAs (spga-lncRNAs)

Two spga-lncRNAs, spga-lncRNA1 and spga-lncRNA2, were identified from a group of (109 single-exonic) lncRNAs that were expressed in type A spermatogonia, pachytene spermatocyte, and round spermatids (Lee et al., 2012). These two spga-lncRNAs were found to be inhibitors of type A spermatogonial differentiation, suggesting a role in maintenance of SSCs.

Narcolepsy Candidate-Region 1 Gene (NLC1-C)

NLC1-C is also known as long intergenic noncoding RNA162 (LINC00162), which is downregulated in the cytoplasm and accumulated in the nucleus of spermatogonia and primary spermatocytes in the testes of infertile men, compared with normal control (Lu et al., 2015). The accumulation of NLC1-C in the nucleus repressed miR-320a and miR-383 transcript and promoted proliferation of testicular embryonic carcinoma cells *in vitro* by binding to nucleolin, indicating that lncRNA NLC1-C modulates miRNA expression at the transcriptional level by binding to RNA-binding proteins to regulate human spermatogenesis (Lu et al., 2015).

Taken together, lncRNAs, unlike sncRNAs, are usually species-specific and less conserved. A large number of lncRNAs have been found, however, their biogenesis and functions for spermatogenesis remain largely unknown.

CONCLUSION

Although much progress has been achieved in the field of male germ cell research, there are still a lot of questions that remain to be answered regarding mammalian spermatogenesis. What signal(s) triggers prospermatogonia transformation to spermatogonia? How is the fate of SSCs determined? How is the differentiation of SSCs regulated? What are the specific molecular markers for SSCs? How do the spermatocytes initiate meiotic division? How is spermiogenesis initiated? What are the molecular mechanisms underlying the degradation of the unnecessary cellular components for sperm function during spermiogenesis? An accumulation of evidence has suggested that the key to address these questions is the understanding of the function of protein coding genes and the regulatory role of ncRNAs during male germ cell development.

Extensive and accurate regulation is required to support the highly orchestrated expression of specific genes required for each step of spermatogenesis. As reviewed in this chapter, a large number and different types of ncRNAs are highly expressed in a stage-specific (or step-specific) manner during spermatogenesis. However, the function of many of those ncRNAs in spermatogenesis is still unknown. In addition to investigation on protein-coding genes (mRNA and proteins) and ncRNAs separately, future studies in the field of male germ cell biology should primarily focus more on integration of the mRNAs/proteins and ncRNAs regulatory networks by a systems biology approach. Since ncRNAs are involved in the transcriptional, posttranscriptional and epigenetic regulation in spermatogenesis, it is essential to study the crosstalk among these different processes in the regulatory network. Secondly, epigenetics has proven to be of paramount importance in the control of gene expression. We predict that future research will become increasingly focused on the understanding of biological functions of epigenetic changes (or marks) during germ cell development. It has been recently discovered that methylation is involved in pri-miRNA processing (Alarcon et al., 2015), opening the door for exploring RNA methylation in the generation and function of ncRNAs. Finally, there will be more types of ncRNAs being discovered in the near future along the annotation of the noncoding sequences in mammalian genomes. It becomes clear that different types of ncRNAs may be related with regard to their biogenesis and function. A good example of this is the tRNA (and/or rRNA)-derived snoRNAs that have a miRNA-like function (Falaleeva and Stamm, 2013), or that act as a subtype of piRNAs to interact with Piwi proteins (Garcia-Lopez et al., 2015). We believe that, in this postgenomics era, it is time for us to explore the noncoding transcriptome of the mammalian genome in every tissue and/or cell type in the body. The annotation of these ncRNAs and the elucidation of their molecular mechanisms during testis development and spermatogenesis will provide insight into the etiology of male sterility and infertility.

Acknowledgments

We would like to thank Dr. Joy Pate for critical review of the manuscript. We also would like to thank Jinzhou Qin, Zhendong Zhu, Jian Du, Xiaoxu Chen, Shuai Yu, Pengfei Zhang and Wuzi Dong in Dr. Wenxian Zeng's laboratory for their help in preparation of figures and for their comments on the draft manuscript. This project is funded, in part, by the National Basic Research Program of China (973 program; No. 2013CB943103), the National Natural Science Foundation of China (No. 31272439, No. 31230048 and No. 31572401), and Programs Foundation of Ministry of Education of China (No. 20130204110017) for WXZ, China Postdoctoral Science Foundation (No.

2014M560809) for CYP, and under a grant with the Huck Institutes of the Life Sciences (at the Pennsylvania State University) and the Pennsylvania Department of Health using Tobacco CURE (Commonwealth Universal Research Enhancement) funds for WSL.

REFERENCES

Agbor, V.A., Tao, S.X., Lei, N., and Heckert, L.L. (2013). A Wt1-Dmrt1 transgene restores DMRT1 to sertoli cells of Dmrt1(-/-) testes: a novel model of DMRT1-Deficient germ cells. *Biol Reprod 88*, 51. doi: 10.1095/biolreprod.112.103135.

Alarcon, C.R., Lee, H., Goodarzi, H., Halberg, N., and Tavazoie, S.F. (2015). N-6-methyladenosine marks primary microRNAs for processing. *Nature 519*, 482-485.

Anguera, M.C., Ma, W.Y., Clift, D., Namekawa, S., Kelleher, R.J., and Lee, J.T. (2011). Tsx produces a long noncoding RNA and has general functions in the germline, Stem Cells, and Brain. *PLoS Genet 7*, e1002248. doi: 10.1371/journal.pgen.1002248.

Aravin, A., Gaidatzis, D., Pfeffer, S., Lagos-Quintana, M., Landgraf, P., Iovino, N., Morris, P., Brownstein, M.J., Kuramochi-Miyagawa, S., and Nakano, T. (2006). A novel class of small RNAs bind to MILI protein in mouse testes. *Nature 442*, 203-207.

Aravin, A.A., Sachidanandam, R., Bourc'his, D., Schaefer, C., Pezic, D., Toth, K.F., Bestor, T., and Hannon, G.J. (2008). A piRNA pathway primed by individual transposons is linked to de novo DNA methylation in mice. *Mol Cell 31*, 785-799.

Aravin, A.A., Sachidanandam, R., Girard, A., Fejes-Toth, K., and Hannon, G.J. (2007). Developmentally regulated piRNA clusters implicate MILI in transposon control. *Science 316*, 744-747.

Aravin, A.A., van der Heijden, G.W., Castaneda, J., Vagin, V.V., Hannon, G.J., and Bortvin, A. (2009). Cytoplasmic compartmentalization of the fetal piRNA pathway in mice. *PLoS Genet 5*, e1000764. doi: 10.1371/journal.pgen.1000764.

Arun, G., Akhade, V.S., Donakonda, S., and Rao, M.R.S. (2012). mrhl RNA, a long noncoding RNA, negatively regulates Wnt signaling through its protein partner Ddx5/p68 in mouse spermatogonial cells. *Mol Cell Biol 32*, 3140-3152.

Bao, J., Wu, J., Schuster, A.S., Hennig, G.W., and Yan, W. (2013). Expression profiling reveals developmentally regulated lncRNA repertoire in the mouse male germline. *Biol Reprod 89*, 107. doi: 10.1095/biolreprod.113.113308.

Bao, J., and Yan, W. (2012). Male germline control of transposable elements. *Biol Reprod 86*, 162, 161-114.

Bao, J.Q., Li, D., Wang, L., Wu, J.W., Hu, Y.Q., Wang, Z.G., Chen, Y., Cao, X.K., Jiang, C.Z., and Yan, W. (2012). MicroRNA-449 and microRNA-34b/c function redundantly in murine testes by targeting E2F transcription factor-retinoblastoma protein (E2F-pRb) pathway. *J Biol Chem 287*, 21686-21698.

Barik, S. (2008). An intronic microRNA silences genes that are functionally antagonistic to its host gene. *Nucleic Acids Res 36*, 5232-5241.

Berghoff, E.G., Clark, M.F., Chen, S., Cajigas, I., Leib, D.E., and Kohtz, J.D. (2013). Evf2 (Dlx6as) lncRNA regulates ultraconserved enhancer methylation and the differential transcriptional control of adjacent genes. *Development 140*, 4407-4416.

Beyret, E., Liu, N., and Lin, H. (2012). piRNA biogenesis during adult spermatogenesis in mice is independent of the ping-pong mechanism. *Cell Res 22*, 1429-1439.

Bjork, J.K., Sandqvist, A., Elsing, A.N., Kotaja, N., and Sistonen, L. (2010). miR-18, a member of Oncomir-1, targets heat shock transcription factor 2 in spermatogenesis. *Development 137*, 3177-3184.

Blow, M.J., Grocock, R.J., van Dongen, S., Enright, A.J., Dicks, E., Futreal, P.A., Wooster, R., and Stratton, M.R. (2006). RNA editing of human microRNAs. *Genome Biol 7*, R27. doi:10.1186/gb-2006-7-4-r27.

Bourc'his, D., and Bestor, T.H. (2004). Meiotic catastrophe and retrotransposon reactivation in male germ cells lacking Dnmt3L. *Nature 431*, 96-99.

Buchold, G.M., Coarfa, C., Kim, J., Milosavljevic, A., Gunaratne, P.H., and Matzuk, M.M. (2010). Analysis of microRNA expression in the prepubertal testis. *PLoS One 5*, e15317. doi: 10.1371/journal.pone.0015317.

Cabili, M.N., Trapnell, C., Goff, L., Koziol, M., Tazon-Vega, B., Regev, A., and Rinn, J.L. (2011). Integrative annotation of human large intergenic noncoding RNAs reveals global properties and specific subclasses. *Genes Dev 25*, 1915-1927.

Cacciola, G., Chioccarelli, T., Fasano, S., Pierantoni, R., and Cobellis, G. (2013). Estrogens and spermiogenesis: new insights from type 1 cannabinoid receptor knockout mice. *Int J Endocrinol 2013*, 501350. doi: 10.1155/2013/501350.

Cai, X.Z., and Cullen, B.R. (2007). The imprinted H19 noncoding RNA is a primary microRNA precursor. *RNA 13*, 313-316.

Cai, X.Z., Hagedorn, C.H., and Cullen, B.R. (2004). Human microRNAs are processed from capped, polyadenylated transcripts that can also function as mRNAs. *RNA 10*, 1957-1966.

Cao, J. (2014). The functional role of long non-coding RNAs and epigenetics. *Biol Proced Online 16*, 11. doi: 10.1186/1480-9222-16-11.

Capel, B., Swain, A., Nicolis, S., Hacker, A., Walter, M., Koopman, P., Goodfellow, P., and Lovell-Badge, R. (1993). Circular transcripts of the testis-determining gene Sry in adult mouse testis. *Cell 73*, 1019-1030.

Castaneda, J., Genzor, P., van der Heijden, G.W., Sarkeshik, A., Yates, J.R., 3rd, Ingolia, N.T., and Bortvin, A. (2014). Reduced pachytene piRNAs and translation underlie spermiogenic arrest in Maelstrom mutant mice. *EMBO J 33*, 1999-2019.

Carlile, M., Swan, D., Jackson, K., Preston-Fayers, K., Ballester, B., Flicek, P., and Werner, A. (2009). Strand selective generation of endo-siRNAs from the Na/phosphate transporter gene Slc34a1 in murine tissues. *Nucleic Acids Res 37*, 2274-2282.

Chalmel, F., Lardenois, A., Evrard, B., Rolland, A.D., Sallou, O., Dumargne, M.C., Coiffec, I., Collin, O., Primig, M., and Jegou, B. (2014). High-resolution profiling of novel transcribed regions during rat spermatogenesis. *Biol Reprod 91*, 5. doi: 10.1095/biolreprod.114.118166.

Chen, C., Jin, J., James, D.A., Adams-Cioaba, M.A., Park, J.G., Guo, Y., Tenaglia, E., Xu, C., Gish, G., and Min, J. (2009). Mouse Piwi interactome identifies binding mechanism of Tdrkh Tudor domain to arginine methylated Miwi. *Proc Natl Acad Sci U S A 106*, 20336-20341.

Chen, T., Hao, Y.J., Zhang, Y., Li, M.M., Wang, M., Han, W.F., Wu, Y.S., Lv, Y., Hao, J., Wang, L.B. et al. (2015). m(6)A RNA methylation is regulated by microRNAs and promotes reprogramming to pluripotency. *Cell Stem Cell 16*, 289-301.

Chuma, S., Hosokawa, M., Kitamura, K., Kasai, S., Fujioka, M., Hiyoshi, M., Takamune, K., Noce, T., and Nakatsuji, N. (2006). Tdrd1/Mtr-1, a tudor-related gene, is essential for male germ-cell differentiation and nuage/germinal granule formation in mice. *Proc Natl Acad Sci U S A 103*, 15894-15899.

Chuma, S., Hosokawa, M., Tanaka, T., and Nakatsuji, N. (2009). Ultrastructural characterization of spermatogenesis and its evolutionary conservation in the germline: germinal granules in mammals. *Mol Cell Endocrinol 306*, 17-23.

Coffey, A.J., Kokocinski, F., Calafato, M.S., Scott, C.E., Palta, P., Drury, E., Joyce, C.J., Leproust, E.M., Harrow, J., Hunt, S. et al. (2011). The GENCODE exome: sequencing the complete human exome. *Eur J Hum Genet: 19*, 827-831.

Czech, B., Malone, C.D., Zhou, R., Stark, A., Schlingeheyde, C., Dus, M., Perrimon, N., Kellis, M., Wohlschlegel, J.A., Sachidanandam, R., Hannon, G.J., and Brennecke, J. (2008). An endogenous small interfering RNA pathway in Drosophila. *Nature 453*, 798- 802.

Dai, L.S., Tsai-Morris, C.H., Sato, H., Villar, J., Kang, J.H., Zhang, J.B., and Dufau, M.L. (2011). Testis-specific miRNA-469 up-regulated in gonadotropin-regulated testicular RNA helicase (GRTH/DDX25)-null mice silences transition protein 2 and protamine 2 messages at sites within coding region: implications of its role in germ cell development. *J Biol Chem 286*, 44306-44318.

Danan, M., Schwartz, S., Edelheit, S., and Sorek, R. (2012). Transcriptome-wide discovery of circular RNAs in Archaea. *Nucleic Acids Res 40*, 3131-3142.

De Fazio, S., Bartonicek, N., Di Giacomo, M., Abreu-Goodger, C., Sankar, A., Funaya, C., Antony, C., Moreira, P.N., Enright, A.J., and O'Carroll, D. (2011). The endonuclease activity of Mili fuels piRNA amplification that silences LINE1 elements. *Nature 480*, 259-263.

de Mateo, S., and Sassone-Corsi, P. (2014). Regulation of spermatogenesis by small non-coding RNAs: role of the germ granule. *Semin Cell Dev Bio*l *29*, 84-92.

de Rooij, D.G., and Russell, L.D. (2000). All you wanted to know about spermatogonia but were afraid to ask. *J Androl 21*, 776-798.

De Santa, F., Barozzi, I., Mietton, F., Ghisletti, S., Polletti, S., Tusi, B.K., Muller, H., Ragoussis, J., Wei, C.L., and Natoli, G. (2010). A large fraction of extragenic RNA pol II transcription sites overlap enhancers. *PLoS Biol 8*, e1000384. doi: 10.1371/journal.pbio.1000384.

Deng, W., and Lin, H.F. (2002). miwi, a murine homolog of piwi, encodes a cytoplasmic protein essential for spermatogenesis. *Dev Cell 2*, 819-830.

Denli, A.M., Tops, B.B.J., Plasterk, R.H.A., Ketting, R.F., and Hannon, G.J. (2004). Processing of primary microRNAs by the Microprocessor complex. *Nature 432*, 231-235.

Derrien, T., Johnson, R., Bussotti, G., Tanzer, A., Djebali, S., Tilgner, H., Guernec, G., Martin, D., Merkel, A., Knowles, D.G. et al. (2012). The

GENCODE v7 catalog of human long noncoding RNAs: Analysis of their gene structure, evolution, and expression. *Genome Res 22*, 1775-1789.

Di Giacomo, M., Comazzetto, S., Saini, H., De Fazio, S., Carrieri, C., Morgan, M., Vasiliauskaite, L., Benes, V., Enright, A.J., and O'Carroll, D. (2013). Multiple epigenetic mechanisms and the piRNA pathway enforce LINE1 silencing during adult spermatogenesis. *Mol Cell 50*, 601-608.

Djebali, S., Davis, C.A., Merkel, A., Dobin, A., Lassmann, T., Mortazavi, A., Tanzer, A., Lagarde, J., Lin, W., Schlesinger, F. et al. (2012). Landscape of transcription in human cells. *Nature 489*, 101-108.

Eddy, E.M. (1975). Germ plasm and the differentiation of the germ cell line. *Int Rev Cytol 43*, 229-280.

Faghihi, M.A., and Wahlestedt, C. (2009). Regulatory roles of natural antisense transcripts. *Nat Rev Mol Cell Biol 10*, 637-643.

Falaleeva, M., and Stamm, S. (2013). Processing of snoRNAs as a new source of regulatory non-coding RNAs: snoRNA fragments form a new class of functional RNAs. *Bioessays 35*, 46-54.

Friedman, R.C., Farh, K.K.H., Burge, C.B., and Bartel, D.P. (2009). Most mammalian mRNAs are conserved targets of microRNAs. *Genome Res 19*, 92-105.

Fu, Q., and Wang, P.J. (2014). Mammalian piRNAs: Biogenesis, function, and mysteries. Spermatogenesis *4*, e27889. eCollection 2014. doi: 10.4161/spmg.27889.

Gan, H., Lin, X., Zhang, Z., Zhang, W., Liao, S., Wang, L., and Han, C. (2011). piRNA profiling during specific stages of mouse spermatogenesis. *RNA 17*, 1191-1203.

Garcia-Lopez, J., Alonso, L., Cardenas, D.B., Artaza-Alvarez, H., Hourcade Jde, D., Martinez, S., Brieno-Enriquez, M.A., and Del Mazo, J. (2015). Diversity and functional convergence of small noncoding RNAs in male germ cell differentiation and fertilization. *RNA 21*, 946-962.

Garcia-Lopez, J., Hourcade Jde, D., Alonso, L., Cardenas, D.B., and del Mazo, J. (2014). Global characterization and target identification of piRNAs and endo-siRNAs in mouse gametes and zygotes. *Biochim Biophys Acta 1839*, 463-475.

Girard, A., Sachidanandam, R., Hannon, G.J., and Carmell, M.A. (2006). A germline-specific class of small RNAs binds mammalian Piwi proteins. *Nature 442*, 199-202.

Goh, W.S., Falciatori, I., Tam, O.H., Burgess, R., Meikar, O., Kotaja, N., Hammell, M., and Hannon, G.J. (2015). piRNA-directed cleavage of meiotic transcripts regulates spermatogenesis. *Genes Dev 29*, 1032-1044.

Gou, L.T., Dai, P., Yang, J.H., Xue, Y., Hu, Y.P., Zhou, Y., Kang, J.Y., Wang, X., Li, H., Hua, M.M. et al. (2014). Pachytene piRNAs instruct massive mRNA elimination during late spermiogenesis. *Cell Res 24*, 680-700.

Gregory, R.I., Yan, K.P., Amuthan, G., Chendrimada, T., Doratotaj, B., Cooch, N., and Shiekhattar, R. (2004). The Microprocessor complex mediates the genesis of microRNAs. *Nature 432*, 235-240.

Grivna, S.T., Beyret, E., Wang, Z., and Lin, H. (2006a). A novel class of small RNAs in mouse spermatogenic cells. *Genes Dev 20*, 1709-1714.

Grivna, S.T., Pyhtila, B., and Lin, H. (2006b). MIWI associates with translational machinery and PIWI-interacting *RNAs* (piRNAs) in regulating spermatogenesis. *Proc Natl Acad Sci U S A 103*, 13415-13420.

Gunawardane, L.S., Saito, K., Nishida, K.M., Miyoshi, K., Kawamura, Y., Nagami, T., Siomi, H., and Siomi, M.C. (2007). A slicer-mediated mechanism for repeat-associated siRNA 5' end formation in Drosophila. *Science 315*, 1587-1590.

Guttman, M., Amit, I., Garber, M., French, C., Lin, M.F., Feldser, D., Huarte, M., Zuk, O., Carey, B.W., Cassady, J.P. et al. (2009). Chromatin signature reveals over a thousand highly conserved large non-coding RNAs in mammals. *Nature 458*, 223-227.

Guzzardo, P.M., Muerdter, F., and Hannon, G.J. (2013). The piRNA pathway in flies: highlights and future directions. *Curr Opin Genet Dev 23*, 44-52.

Ha, H., Song, J., Wang, S., Kapusta, A., Feschotte, C., Chen, K.C., and Xing, J. (2014). A comprehensive analysis of piRNAs from adult human testis and their relationship with genes and mobile elements. *BMC Genomics 15*, 545. doi: 10.1186/1471-2164-15-545.

Ha, M., and Kim, V.N. (2014). Regulation of microRNA biogenesis. *Nat Rev Mol Cell Bio 15*, 509-524.

Han, J.J., Lee, Y., Yeom, K.H., Kim, Y.K., Jin, H., and Kim, V.N. (2004). The Drosha-DGCR8 complex in primary microRNA processing. *Genes Dev 18*, 3016-3027.

Hansen, T.B., Jensen, T.I., Clausen, B.H., Bramsen, J.B., Finsen, B., Damgaard, C.K., and Kjems, J. (2013). Natural RNA circles function as efficient microRNA sponges. *Nature 495*, 384-388.

Harrow, J., Frankish, A., Gonzalez, J.M., Tapanari, E., Diekhans, M., Kokocinski, F., Aken, B.L., Barrell, D., Zadissa, A., Searle, S. et al. (2012). GENCODE: the reference human genome annotation for The ENCODE Project. *Genome Res 22*, 1760-1774.

Hata, K., Okano, M., Lei, H., and Li, E. (2002). Dnmt3L cooperates with the Dnmt3 family of de novo DNA methyltransferases to establish maternal imprints in mice. *Development 129*, 1983-1993.

Hayashi, K., Lopes, S.M.C.D., Kaneda, M., Tang, F.C., Hajkova, P., Lao, K.Q., O'Carroll, D., Das, P.P., Tarakhovsky, A., Miska, E.A. et al. (2008). MicroRNA Biogenesis Is Required for Mouse Primordial Germ Cell Development and Spermatogenesis. *PLoS One 3*, e1738. doi: 10.1371/journal.pone.0001738.

He, Z., Kokkinaki, M., Pant, D., Gallicano, G.I., Dym, M. (2009). Small RNA molecules in the regulation of spermatogenesis. *Reproduction 137*, 901-911.

He, Z.P., Jiang, J.J., Kokkinaki, M., Tang, L., Zeng, W.X., Gallicano, I., Dobrinski, I., and Dym, M. (2013). MiRNA-20 and miRNA-106a regulate spermatogonial stem cell renewal at the post-transcriptional level via targeting STAT3 and Ccnd1. *Stem Cells 31*, 2205-2217.

Hermo, L., Pelletier, R.M., Cyr, D.G., and Smith, C.E. (2010a). Surfing the wave, cycle, life history, and genes/proteins expressed by testicular germ cells. Part 1: background to spermatogenesis, spermatogonia, and spermatocytes. *Microsc Res Tech 73*, 241-278.

Hermo, L., Pelletier, R.M., Cyr, D.G., and Smith, C.E. (2010b). Surfing the wave, cycle, life history, and genes/proteins expressed by testicular germ cells. Part 2: changes in spermatid organelles associated with development of spermatozoa. *Microsc Res Tech 73*, 279-319.

Hermo, L., Pelletier, R.M., Cyr, D.G., and Smith, C.E. (2010c). Surfing the wave, cycle, life history, and genes/proteins expressed by testicular germ cells. Part 3: developmental changes in spermatid flagellum and cytoplasmic droplet and interaction of sperm with the zona pellucida and egg plasma membrane. *Microsc Res Tech 73*, 320-363.

Hermo, L., Pelletier, R.M., Cyr, D.G., and Smith, C.E. (2010d). Surfing the wave, cycle, life history, and genes/proteins expressed by testicular germ cells. Part 4: intercellular bridges, mitochondria, nuclear envelope, apoptosis, ubiquitination, membrane/voltage-gated channels, methylation/acetylation, and transcription factors. *Microsc Res Tech 73*, 364-408.

Hermo, L., Pelletier, R.M., Cyr, D.G., and Smith, C.E. (2010e). Surfing the Wave, Cycle, Life History, and Genes/Proteins Expressed by Testicular Germ Cells. Part 5: Intercellular Junctions and Contacts Between Germs Cells and Sertoli Cells and Their Regulatory Interactions, Testicular

Cholesterol, and Genes/Proteins Associated With More Than One Germ Cell Generation. *Microsc Res Techniq 73*, 409-494.

Hirano, T., Iwasaki, Y.W., Lin, Z.Y., Imamura, M., Seki, N.M., Sasaki, E., Saito, K., Okano, H., Siomi, M.C., and Siomi, H. (2014). Small RNA profiling and characterization of piRNA clusters in the adult testes of the common marmoset, a model primate. *RNA 20*, 1223-1237.

Houwing, S., Kamminga, L.M., Berezikov, E., Cronembold, D., Girard, A., van den Elst, H., Filippov, D.V., Blaser, H., Raz, E., Moens, C.B. et al. (2007). A role for Piwi and piRNAs in germ cell maintenance and transposon silencing in Zebrafish. *Cell 129*, 69-82.

Hsu, M.T., and Coca-Prados, M. (1979). Electron microscopic evidence for the circular form of RNA in the cytoplasm of eukaryotic cells. *Nature 280*, 339-340.

Hua, J. (2015). miR-204 regulated the proliferation of dairy goat spermatogonial stem cells via targeting to Sirt1. *Rejuvenation Res.* [Epub ahead of print] (URL: http://www.ncbi.nlm.nih.gov/pubmed/26213858)

Hung, T., Wang, Y.L., Lin, M.F., Koegel, A.K., Kotake, Y., Grant, G.D., Horlings, H.M., Shah, N., Umbricht, C., Wang, P. et al. (2011). Extensive and coordinated transcription of noncoding RNAs within cell-cycle promoters. *Nat Genet 43*, 621-629.

Huszar, J.M., and Payne, C.J. (2013). MicroRNA 146 (Mir146) modulates spermatogonial differentiation by retinoic acid in mice. *Biol Reprod 88*, 15. doi: 10.1095/biolreprod.112.103747.

Jalali, S., Bhartiya, D., Lalwani, M.K., Sivasubbu, S., and Scaria, V. (2013). Systematic transcriptome wide analysis of lncRNA-miRNA interactions. *PLoS One 8*, e53823. doi: 10.1371/journal.pone.0053823.

Jeck, W.R., Sorrentino, J.A., Wang, K., Slevin, M.K., Burd, C.E., Liu, J., Marzluff, W.F., and Sharpless, N.E. (2013). Circular RNAs are abundant, conserved, and associated with ALU repeats. *RNA 19*, 141-157.

Kim, T.K., Hemberg, M., Gray, J.M., Costa, A.M., Bear, D.M., Wu, J., Harmin, D.A., Laptewicz, M., Barbara-Haley, K., Kuersten, S. et al. (2010). Widespread transcription at neuronal activity-regulated enhancers. *Nature 465*, 182-187.

Kimmins, S., and Sassone-Corsi, P. (2005). Chromatin remodelling and epigenetic features of germ cells. *Nature 434*, 583-589.

Klattenhoff, C., Bratu, D.P., McGinnis-Schultz, N., Koppetsch, B.S., Cook, H.A., and Theurkauf, W.E. (2007). Drosophila rasiRNA pathway mutations disrupt embryonic axis specification through activation of an ATR/Chk2 DNA damage response. *Dev Cell 12*, 45-55.

Kolakofsky, D. (1976). Isolation and characterization of Sendai virus DI-RNAs. *Cell 8*, 547-555.

Kraus, P., Sivakamasundari, V., Lim, S.L., Xing, X., Lipovich, L., and Lufkin, T. (2013). Making sense of Dlx1 antisense RNA. *Dev Biol 376*, 224-235.

Krol, J., Loedige, I., and Filipowicz, W. (2010). The widespread regulation of microRNA biogenesis, function and decay. *Nat Rev Genet 11*, 597-610.

Kuramochi-Miyagawa, S., Watanabe, T., Gotoh, K., Totoki, Y., Toyoda, A., Ikawa, M., Asada, N., Kojima, K., Yamaguchi, Y., Ijiri, T.W. et al. (2008). DNA methylation of retrotransposon genes is regulated by Piwi family members MILI and MIWI2 in murine fetal testes. *Genes Dev 22*, 908-917.

Kotaja, N. (2014). MicroRNAs and spermatogenesis. *Fertil Steril 101*, 1552-1562.

Kutter, C., Watt, S., Stefflova, K., Wilson, M.D., Goncalves, A., Ponting, C.P., Odom, D.T., and Marques, A.C. (2012). Rapid turnover of long noncoding RNAs and the evolution of gene expression. *PLoS Genet 8*, e1002841. doi: 10.1371/journal.pgen.1002841.

Lagos-Quintana, M., Rauhut, R., Lendeckel, W., and Tuschl, T. (2001). Identification of novel genes coding for small expressed RNAs. *Science 294*, 853-858.

Laiho, A., Kotaja, N., Gyenesei, A., and Sironen, A. (2013). Transcriptome profiling of the murine testis during the first wave of spermatogenesis. *PLoS One 8*, e61558. doi: 10.1371/journal.pone.0061558.

Landthaler, M., Yalcin, A., and Tuschl, T. (2004). The human DiGeorge syndrome critical region gene 8 and its D-melanogaster homolog are required for miRNA biogenesis. *Curr Biol 14*, 2162-2167.

Lau, N.C., Lim, L.P., Weinstein, E.G., and Bartel, D.P. (2001). An abundant class of tiny RNAs with probable regulatory roles in Caenorhabditis elegans. *Science 294*, 858-862.

Lee, R.C., and Ambros, V. (2001). An extensive class of small RNAs in Caenorhabditis elegans. *Science 294*, 862-864.

Lee, T.L., Pang, A.L., Rennert, O.M., and Chan, W.Y. (2009). Genomic landscape of developing male germ cells. *Birth Defects Res C Embryo Today 87*, 43-63.

Lee, T.L., Xiao, A., and Rennert, O.M. (2012). Identification of novel long noncoding RNA transcripts in male germ cells. *Methods Mol Biol 825*, 105-114.

Lee, Y., Ahn, C., Han, J.J., Choi, H., Kim, J., Yim, J., Lee, J., Provost, P., Radmark, O., Kim, S. et al. (2003). The nuclear RNase III Drosha initiates microRNA processing. *Nature 425*, 415-419.

Lee, Y., Hur, I., Park, S.Y., Kim, Y.K., Suh, M.R., and Kim, V.N. (2006). The role of PACT in the RNA silencing pathway. *EMBO J 25*, 522-532.

Lee, Y., Kim, M., Han, J.J., Yeom, K.H., Lee, S., Baek, S.H., and Kim, V.N. (2004). MicroRNA genes are transcribed by RNA polymerase II. *EMBO J* 23, 4051-4060.

Lewis, B.P., Burge, C.B., and Bartel, D.P. (2005). Conserved seed pairing, often flanked by adenosines, indicates that thousands of human genes are microRNA targets. *Cell 120*, 15-20.

Li, M., Yu, M., Liu, C., Zhu, H., He, X., Peng, S., and Hua, J. (2013). miR-34c works downstream of p53 leading to dairy goat male germline stem-cell (mGSCs) apoptosis. *Cell Prolif 46*, 223-231.

Liang, M., Li, W.Q., Tian, H., Hu, T., Wang, L., Lin, Y., Li, Y.L., Huang, H.F., and Sun, F. (2014). Sequential expression of long noncoding RNA as mRNA gene expression in specific stages of mouse spermatogenesis. *Sci Rep 4*, 5966. doi: 10.1038/srep05966.

Liang, X.X., Zhou, D.D., Wei, C., Luo, H.S., Liu, J.L., Fu, R., and Cui, S. (2012). MicroRNA-34c enhances murine male germ cell apoptosis through targeting ATF1. *PLoS One 7*, e33861. doi: 10.1371/journal.pone.0033861.

Lim, S.L., Qu, Z.P., Kortschak, R.D., Lawrence, D.M., Geoghegan, J., Hempfling, A.L., Bergmann, M., Goodnow, C.C., Ormandy, C.J., Wong, L. et al. (2015). HENMT1 and piRNA stability are required for adult male germ cell transposon repression and to define the spermatogenic program in the mouse. *PLoS Genet 11*, e1005620. doi: 10.1371/journal.pgen.1005620.

Lin, H. (2007). piRNAs in the germ line. *Science 316*, 397.

Liu, Y., Niu, M.H., Yao, C.C., Hai, Y.N., Yuan, Q.Q., Liu, Y., Guo, Y., Li, Z., and He, Z.P. (2015). Fractionation of human spermatogenic cells using STA-PUT gravity sedimentation and their miRNA profiling. *Sci Rep 5*, 8084. doi: 10.1038/srep08084.

Lu, M., Tian, H., Cao, Y.X., He, X., Chen, L., Song, X., Ping, P., Huang, H., and Sun, F. (2015). Downregulation of miR-320a/383-sponge-like long non-coding RNA NLC1-C (narcolepsy candidate-region 1 genes) is associated with male infertility and promotes testicular embryonal carcinoma cell proliferation. *Cell Death Dis 6*, e1960. doi: 10.1038/cddis.2015.267.

Luk, A.C., Chan, W.Y., Rennert, O.M., and Lee, T.L. (2014). Long noncoding RNAs in spermatogenesis: insights from recent high-throughput transcriptome studies. *Reproduction 147*, R131-R141. doi: 10.1530/REP-13-0594.

Lund, E., Guttinger, S., Calado, A., Dahlberg, J.E., and Kutay, U. (2004). Nuclear export of microRNA precursors. *Science 303*, 95-98.

Luo, Z.G., Liu, Y.K., Chen, L., Ellis, M., Li, M.Z., Wang, J.Y., Zhang, Y., Fu, P.H., Wang, K.T., Li, X.W. et al. (2015). microRNA profiling in three main stages during porcine spermatogenesis. *J Assist Reprod Genet 32*, 451-460.

Ma, L., Buchold, G.M., Greenbaum, M.P., Roy, A., Burns, K.H., Zhu, H., Han, D.Y., Harris, R.A., Coarfa, C., Gunaratne, P.H. et al. (2009). GASZ is essential for male meiosis and suppression of retrotransposon expression in the male germline. *PLoS Genet 5*, e1000635. doi: 10.1371/journal.pgen.1000635.

Marchese, F.P., and Huarte, M. (2014). Long non-coding RNAs and chromatin modifiers: their place in the epigenetic code. *Epigenetics 9*, 21-26.

Marcon, E., Babak, T., Chua, G., Hughes, T., and Moens, P.B. (2008). miRNA and piRNA localization in the male mammalian meiotic nucleus. *Chromosome Res 16*, 243-260.

Martinez, J., and Tuschl, T. (2004). RISC is a 5 ' phosphomonoester-producing RNA endonuclease. *Genes Dev 18*, 975-980.

Marushige, K., and Dixon, G.H. (1969). Developmental changes in chromosomal composition and template activity during spermatogenesis in trout testis. *Dev Biol 19*, 397-414.

McIver, S.C., Roman, S.D., Nixon, B., and McLaughlin, E.A. (2012a). miRNA and mammalian male germ cells. *Hum Reprod Update 18*, 44-59.

McIver, S.C., Stanger, S.J., Santarelli, D.M., Roman, S.D., Nixon, B., and McLaughlin, E.A. (2012b). A unique combination of male germ cell miRNAs coordinates gonocyte differentiation. *PLoS One 7* e35553. doi: 10.1371/journal.pone.0035553.

Meikar, O., Da Ros, M., Korhonen, H., and Kotaja, N. (2011). Chromatoid body and small RNAs in male germ cells. *Reproduction 142*, 195-209.

Meikar, O., Da Ros, M., and Kotaja, N. (2013). Epigenetic regulation of male germ cell differentiation. *Subcell Biochem 61*, 119-138.

Meister, G., and Tuschl, T. (2004). Mechanisms of gene silencing by double-stranded RNA. *Nature 431*, 343-349.

Memczak, S., Jens, M., Elefsinioti, A., Torti, F., Krueger, J., Rybak, A., Maier, L., Mackowiak, S.D., Gregersen, L.H., Munschauer, M. et al.

(2013). Circular RNAs are a large class of animal RNAs with regulatory potency. *Nature 495*, 333-338.

Mirkovic-Hosle, M., and Forstemann, K. (2014). Transposon defense by endo-siRNAs, piRNAs and somatic pilRNAs in Drosophila: contributions of Loqs-PD and R2D2. *PLoS One 9*, e84994. doi: 10.1371/journal.pone.0084994.

Moritoki, Y., Hayashi, Y., Mizuno, K., Kamisawa, H., Nishio, H., Kurokawa, S., Ugawa, S., Kojima, Y., and Kohri, K. (2014). Expression profiling of microRNA in cryptorchid testes: miR-135a contributes to the maintenance of spermatogonial stem cells by regulating FoxO1. *J Urol 191*, 1174-1180.

Morris, K.V., Chan, S.W., Jacobsen, S.E., and Looney, D.J. (2004). Small interfering RNA-induced transcriptional gene silencing in human cells. *Science 305*, 1289-1292.

Mukherjee, A., Koli, S., and Reddy, K.V.R. (2014). Regulatory non-coding transcripts in spermatogenesis: shedding light on 'dark matter.' *Andrology 2*, 360-369.

Ng, S.Y., Bogu, G.K., Soh, B.S., and Stanton, L.W. (2013). The long noncoding RNA RMST interacts with SOX2 to regulate neurogenesis. *Mol Cell 51*, 349-359.

Ni, M.J., Hu, Z.H., Liu, Q., Liu, M.F., Lu, M.H., Zhang, J.S., Zhang, L., and Zhang, Y.L. (2011). Identification and characterization of a novel non-coding RNA involved in sperm maturation. *PLoS One 6* e26053. doi: 10.1371/journal.pone.0026053.

Niu, Z.Y., Goodyear, S.M., Rao, S., Wu, X., Tobias, J.W., Avarbock, M.R., and Brinster, R.L. (2011). MicroRNA-21 regulates the self-renewal of mouse spermatogonial stem cells. *Proc Natl Acad Sci U S A 108*, 12740-12745.

Novotny, G.W., Sonne, S.B., Nielsen, J.E., Jonstrup, S.P., Hansen, M.A., Skakkebaek, N.E., Rajpert-De Meyts, E., Kjems, J., and Leffers, H. (2007). Translational repression of E2F1 mRNA in carcinoma in situ and normal testis correlates with expression of the miR-17-92 cluster. *Cell Death Differ Cell 14*, 879-882.

Oakberg, E.F. (1956). Duration of spermatogenesis in the mouse and timing of stages of the cycle of the seminiferous epithelium. *Am J Anat 99*, 507-516.

Ottolenghi, C., Veitia, R., Barbieri, M., Fellous, M., and McElreavey, K. (2000). The human doublesex-related gene, DMRT2 is homologous to a gene involved in somitogenesis and encodes a potential bicistronic transcript. *Genomics 64*, 179-186.

Papaioannou, M.D., and Nef, S. (2010). microRNAs in the testis: building up male fertility. *J Androl 31*, 26-33.

Paronetto, M.P., and Sette, C. (2010). Role of RNA-binding proteins in mammalian spermatogenesis. *Int J Androl 33*, 2-12.

Pauli, A., Valen, E., Lin, M.F., Garber, M., Vastenhouw, N.L., Levin, J.Z., Fan, L., Sandelin, A., Rinn, J.L., Regev, A. et al. (2012). Systematic identification of long noncoding RNAs expressed during zebrafish embryogenesis. *Genome Res 22*, 577-591.

Phillips, B.T., Gassei, K., and Orwig, K.E. (2010). Spermatogonial stem cell regulation and spermatogenesis. *Philos Trans R Soc Lond B Biol Sci 365*, 1663-1678.

Qin, D., Huang, L., Wlodaver, A., Andrade, J., and Staley, J.P. (2015). Sequencing of lariat termini in S. cerevisiae reveals 5' splice sites, branch points, and novel splicing events. *RNA*. [Epub ahead of print] (URL: http://www.ncbi.nlm.nih.gov/pubmed/26647463).

Quek, X.C., Thomson, D.W., Maag, J.L., Bartonicek, N., Signal, B., Clark, M.B., Gloss, B.S., and Dinger, M.E. (2015). lncRNAdb v2.0: expanding the reference database for functional long noncoding *RNAs. Nucleic Acids Res 43*, D168-D173. doi: 10.1093/nar/gku988.

Rathke, C., Baarends, W.M., Awe, S., and Renkawitz-Pohl, R. (2014). Chromatin dynamics during spermiogenesis. *Biochim Biophys Acta 1839*, 155-168.

Reuter, M., Berninger, P., Chuma, S., Shah, H., Hosokawa, M., Funaya, C., Antony, C., Sachidanandam, R., and Pillai, R.S. (2011). Miwi catalysis is required for piRNA amplification-independent LINE1 transposon silencing. *Nature 480*, 264-267.

Rinn, J.L., and Chang, H.Y. (2012). Genome regulation by long noncoding RNAs. *Annu Rev Biochem 81*, 145-166.

Ro, S., Park, C., Sanders, K.M., McCarrey, J.R., and Yan, W. (2007). Cloning and expression profiling of testis-expressed microRNAs. *Dev Biol 311*, 592-602.

Saito, K., Sakaguchi, Y., Suzuki, T., Suzuki, T., Siomi, H., and Siomi, M.C. (2007). Pimet, the Drosophila homolog of HEN1, mediates 2'-O-methylation of Piwi- interacting RNAs at their 3' ends. *Genes Dev 21*, 1603-1608.

Salzman, J., Gawad, C., Wang, P.L., Lacayo, N., and Brown, P.O. (2012). Circular RNAs are the predominant transcript isoform from hundreds of human genes in diverse cell types. *PLoS One 7*, e30733. doi: 10.1371/ journal.pone.0030733.

Sasaki, T., Shiohama, A., Minoshima, S., and Shimizu, N. (2003). Identification of eight members of the Argonaute family in the human genome. *Genomics 82*, 323-330.

Saxe, J.P., Chen, M., Zhao, H., and Lin, H. (2013). Tdrkh is essential for spermatogenesis and participates in primary piRNA biogenesis in the germline. *EMBO J 32*, 1869-1885.

Schaefer, C.B., Ooi, S.K., Bestor, T.H., and Bourc'his, D. (2007). Epigenetic decisions in mammalian germ cells. *Science 316*, 398-399.

Schulz, R.W., and Miura, T. (2002). Spermatogenesis and its endocrine regulation. *Fish Physiol Biochem 26*, 43-56.

Shima, J.E., McLean, D.J., McCarrey, J.R., and Griswold, M.D. (2004). The murine testicular transcriptome: characterizing gene expression in the testis during the progression of spermatogenesis. *Biol Reprod 71*, 319-330.

Shoji, M., Tanaka, T., Hosokawa, M., Reuter, M., Stark, A., Kato, Y., Kondoh, G., Okawa, K., Chujo, T., Suzuki, T. et al. (2009). The TDRD9-MIWI2 complex is essential for piRNA-mediated retrotransposon silencing in the mouse male germline. *Dev Cell 17*, 775-787.

Siomi, M.C., Sato, K., Pezic, D., and Aravin, A.A. (2011). PIWI-interacting small RNAs: the vanguard of genome defence. *Nat Rev Mol Cell Biol 12*, 246-258.

Smorag, L., Zheng, Y., Nolte, J., Zechner, U., Engel, W., and Pantakani, D.V.K. (2012). MicroRNA signature in various cell types of mouse spermatogenesis: Evidence for stage-specifically expressed miRNA-221, -203 and -34b-5p mediated spermatogenesis regulation. *Biol Cell 104*, 677-692.

Song, J.J., Smith, S.K., Hannon, G.J., and Joshua-Tor, L. (2004). Crystal structure of Argonaute and its implications for RISC slicer activity. *Science 305*, 1434-1437.

Song, R., Hennig, G.W., Wu, Q., Jose, C., Zheng, H., and Yan, W. (2011). Male germ cells express abundant endogenous siRNAs. *Proc Natl Acad Sci USA 108*, 13159-13164.

Song, W.C., Mu, H.L., Wu, J., Liao, M.Z., Zhu, H.J., Zheng, L.M., He, X., Niu, B.W., Zhai, Y.X., Bai, C.L. et al. (2015). miR-544 Regulates Dairy Goat Male Germline Stem Cell Self-Renewal via Targeting PLZF. *J Cell Biochem 116*, 2155-2165.

Sood, P., Krek, A., Zavolan, M., Macino, G., and Rajewsky, N. (2006). Cell-type-specific signatures of microRNAs on target mRNA expression. *Proc Natl Acad Sci U S A 103*, 2746-2751.

Soper, S.F., van der Heijden, G.W., Hardiman, T.C., Goodheart, M., Martin, S.L., de Boer, P., and Bortvin, A. (2008). Mouse maelstrom, a component of nuage, is essential for spermatogenesis and transposon repression in meiosis. *Dev Cell 15*, 285-297.

Suh, N., and Blelloch, R. (2011). Small RNAs in early mammalian development: from gametes to gastrulation. *Development 138*, 1653-1661.

Sun, J., Lin, Y., and Wu, J. (2013). Long non-coding RNA expression profiling of mouse testis during postnatal development. *PLoS One 8*, e75750. doi: 10.1371/journal.pone.0075750.

Sun, J., and Wu, J. (2015). Expression profiling of long noncoding RNAs in neonatal and adult mouse testis. *Data Brief 4*, 322-327.

Tam, O.H., Aravin, A.A., Stein, P., Girard, A., Murchison, E.P., Cheloufi, S., Hodges, E., Anger, M., Sachidanandam, R., Schultz, R.M. et al. (2008). Pseudogene-derived small interfering RNAs regulate gene expression in mouse oocytes. *Nature 453*, 534-538.

Tan, T., Zhang, Y., Ji, W., and Zheng, P. (2014). miRNA signature in mouse spermatogonial stem cells revealed by high-throughput sequencing. *Biomed Res Int 2014*, 154251. doi: 10.1155/2014/154251.

Tong, M.H., Mitchell, D., Evanoff, R., and Griswold, M.D. (2011). Expression of Mirlet7 family microRNAs in response to retinoic acid-induced spermatogonial differentiation in mice. *Biol Reprod 85*, 189-197.

Tong, M.H., Mitchell, D.A., McGowan, S.D., Evanoff, R., and Griswold, M.D. (2012). Two miRNA clusters, Mir-17-92 (Mirc1) and Mir-106b-25 (Mirc3), are involved in the regulation of spermatogonial differentiation in mice. *Biol Reprod 86*, 72. doi: 10.1095/biolreprod.111.096313.

Truscott, M., Islam, A.B., and Frolov, M.V. (2016). Novel regulation and functional interaction of polycistronic miRNAs. *RNA 22*, 129-138.

Ulitsky, I., and Bartel, D.P. (2013). lincRNAs: genomics, evolution, and mechanisms. *Cell 154*, 26-46.

Unhavaithaya, Y., Hao, Y., Beyret, E., Yin, H., Kuramochi-Miyagawa, S., Nakano, T., and Lin, H. (2009). MILI, a PIWI-interacting RNA-binding protein, is required for germ line stem cell self-renewal and appears to positively regulate translation. *J Biol Chem 284*, 6507-6519.

Vagin, V.V., Sigova, A., Li, C., Seitz, H., Gvozdev, V., and Zamore, P.D. (2006). A distinct small RNA pathway silences selfish genetic elements in the germline. *Science 313*, 320-324.

van Bakel, H., Nislow, C., Blencowe, B.J., and Hughes, T.R. (2010). Most "dark matter" transcripts are associated with known genes. *PLoS Biol 8*, e1000371. doi: 10.1371/journal.pbio.1000371.

Villegas, V.E., and Zaphiropoulos, P.G. (2015). Neighboring gene regulation by antisense long non-coding RNAs. *Int J Mol Sci 16*, 3251-3266.

Vourekas, A., Zheng, Q., Alexiou, P., Maragkakis, M., Kirino, Y., Gregory, B.D., and Mourelatos, Z. (2012). Mili and Miwi target RNA repertoire reveals piRNA biogenesis and function of Miwi in spermiogenesis. *Nat Struct Mol Biol 19*, 773-781.

Waclawska, A., and Kurpisz, M. (2012). Key functional genes of spermatogenesis identified by microarray analysis. *Syst Biol Reprod Med 58*, 229-235.

Wang, Y., Li, Y., Toth, J.I., Petroski, M.D., Zhang, Z.L., and Zhao, J.C. (2014). N-6-methyladenosine modification destabilizes developmental regulators in embryonic stem cells. *Nat Cell Biol 16*, 191-198.

Wang, L., and Xu, C. (2015). Role of microRNAs in mammalian spermatogenesis and testicular germ cell tumors. *Reproduction 149*, R127-R137. doi: 10.1530/REP-14-0239.

Wapinski, O., and Chang, H.Y. (2011). Long noncoding RNAs and human disease. *Trends Cell Biol 21*, 354-361.

Wasik, K.A., Tam, O.H., Knott, S.R., Falciatori, I., Hammell, M., Vagin, V.V., and Hannon, G.J. (2015). RNF17 blocks promiscuous activity of PIWI proteins in mouse testes. *Genes Dev 29*, 1403-1415.

Watanabe, T., Cheng, E.C., Zhong, M., and Lin, H. (2015). Retrotransposons and pseudogenes regulate mRNAs and lncRNAs via the piRNA pathway in the germline. *Genome Res 25*, 368-380.

Watanabe, T., Chuma, S., Yamamoto, Y., Kuramochi-Miyagawa, S., Totoki, Y., Toyoda, A., Hoki, Y., Fujiyama, A., Shibata, T., Sado, T. et al. (2011a). MITOPLD is a mitochondrial protein essential for nuage formation and piRNA biogenesis in the mouse germline. *Dev Cell 20*, 364-375.

Watanabe, T., Tomizawa, S., Mitsuya, K., Totoki, Y., Yamamoto, Y., Kuramochi-Miyagawa, S., Iida, N., Hoki, Y., Murphy, P.J., Toyoda, A. et al. (2011b). Role for piRNAs and noncoding RNA in de novo DNA methylation of the imprinted mouse Rasgrf1 locus. *Science 332*, 848-852.

Wen, J., Duan, H., Bejarano, F., Okamura, K., Fabian, L., Brill, J.A., Bortolamiol-Becet, D., Martin, R., Ruby, J.G., and Lai, E.C. (2015). Adaptive regulation of testis gene expression and control of male fertility by the Drosophila hairpin RNA pathway. *Mol Cell 57*, 165-178.

Wu, J., Liao, M.Z., Zhu, H.J., Kang, K., Mu, H.L., Song, W.C., Niu, Z.W., He, X., Bai, C.L., Li, G.P. et al. (2014a). CD49f-positive testicular cells in saanen dairy goat were identified as spermatogonia-like cells by miRNA profiling analysis. *J Cell Biochem 115*, 1712-1723.

Wu, J.W., Bao, J.Q., Kim, M., Yuan, S.Q., Tang, C., Zheng, H.L., Mastick, G.S., Xu, C., and Yan, W. (2014b). Two miRNA clusters, miR-34b/c and miR-449, are essential for normal brain development, motile ciliogenesis, and spermatogenesis. *Proc Natl Acad Sci USA 111*, E2851-E2857. doi: 10.1073/pnas.1407777111.

Wu, Q., Song, R., Ortogero, N., Zheng, H., Evanoff, R., Small, C.L., Griswold, M.D., Namekawa, S.H., Royo, H., Turner, J.M. et al. (2012). The RNase III enzyme DROSHA is essential for microRNA production and spermatogenesis. *J Biol Chem 287*, 25173-25190.

Yadav, R.P., and Kotaja, N. (2014). Small RNAs in spermatogenesis. *Mol Cell Endocrinol 382*, 498-508.

Yan, N.H., Lu, Y.L., Sun, H.Q., Tao, D.C., Zhang, S.Z., Liu, W.Y., and Ma, Y.X. (2007). A microarray for microRNA profiling in mouse testis tissues. *Reproduction 134*, 73-79.

Yao, C., Liu, Y., Sun, M., Niu, M., Yuan, Q., Hai, Y., Guo, Y., Chen, Z., Hou, J., Liu, Y. et al. (2015). MicroRNAs and DNA methylation as epigenetic regulators of mitosis, meiosis and spermiogenesis. *Reproduction 150*, R25-R34. doi: 10.1530/REP-14-0643.

Yi, R., Qin, Y., Macara, I.G., and Cullen, B.R. (2003). Exportin-5 mediates the nuclear export of pre-microRNAs and short hairpin RNAs. *Genes Dev 17*, 3011-3016.

Yin, Q.F., Yang, L., Zhang, Y., Xiang, J.F., Wu, Y.W., Carmichael, G.G., and Chen, L.L. (2012). Long noncoding RNAs with snoRNA ends. *Mol Cell 48*, 219-230.

Yu, Z.R., Raabe, T., and Hecht, N.B. (2005). MicroRNA Mirn122a reduces expression of the posttranscriptionally regulated germ cell transition protein 2 (Tnp2) messenger RNA (mRNA) by mRNA cleavage. *Biol Reprod 73*, 427-433.

Zhang, L., Lu, H., Xin, D., Cheng, H., and Zhou, R. (2010). A novel ncRNA gene from mouse chromosome 5 trans-splices with Dmrt1 on chromosome 19. *Biochem Biophys Res Commun 400*, 696-700.

Zhang, P., Kang, J.Y., Gou, L.T., Wang, J., Xue, Y., Skogerboe, G., Dai, P., Huang, D.W., Chen, R., Fu, X.D. et al. (2015). MIWI and piRNA-mediated cleavage of messenger RNAs in mouse testes. *Cell Res 25*, 193-207.

Zhang, Y., Yang, L., and Chen, L.L. (2014). Life without A tail: new formats of long noncoding RNAs. *Int J Biochem Cell Biol 54*, 338-349.

Zhang, Y., Zhang, X.O., Chen, T., Xiang, J.F., Yin, Q.F., Xing, Y.H., Zhu, S., Yang, L., and Chen, L.L. (2013). Circular intronic long noncoding RNAs. *Mol Cell 51*, 792-806.

Zhao, S., Gou, L.T., Zhang, M., Zu, L.D., Hua, M.M., Hua, Y., Shi, H.J., Li, Y., Li, J., Li, D. et al. (2013). piRNA-triggered MIWI ubiquitination and removal by APC/C in late spermatogenesis. *Dev Cell 24*, 13-25.

Zheng, K., and Wang, P.J. (2012). Blockade of pachytene piRNA biogenesis reveals a novel requirement for maintaining post-meiotic germline genome integrity. *PLoS Genet 8*, e1003038. doi: 10.1371/journal. pgen.1003038.

Zheng, K., Xiol, J., Reuter, M., Eckardt, S., Leu, N.A., McLaughlin, K.J., Stark, A., Sachidanandam, R., Pillai, R.S., and Wang, P.J. (2010). Mouse MOV10L1 associates with Piwi proteins and is an essential component of the Piwi-interacting RNA (piRNA) pathway. *Proc Natl Acad Sci U S A 107*, 11841-11846.

Zhou, R., Czech, B., Brennecke, J., Sachidanandam, R., Wohlschlegel, J.A., Perrimon, N., and Hannon, G.J. (2009). Processing of Drosophila endo-siRNAs depends on a specific Loquacious isoform. *RNA 15*, 1886-1895.

Zimmermann, C., Romero, Y., Warnefors, M., Bilican, A., Borel, C., Smith, L.B., Kotaja, N., Kaessmann, H., and Nef, S. (2014). Germ cell-specific targeting of DICER or DGCR8 reveals a novel role for endo-siRNAs in the progression of mammalian spermatogenesis and male fertility. *PLoS One 9*, e107023. doi: 10.1371/journal.pone.0107023.

In: Spermatogenesis
Editor: Gladys Robinson

ISBN: 978-1-63484-715-5

Chapter 3

TESTICULAR IMMUNE ENVIRONMENT FOR SPERMATOGENESIS

Tingting Deng[1] and Daishu Han[2,*]

[1]Institute of Clinical Medical Sciences,
China-Japan Friendship Hospital, Beijing, China
[2]Department of Cell Biology, Institute of Basic Medical Sciences,
Chinese Academy of Medical Sciences,
School of Basic Medicine, Peking Union Medical College,
Beijing, China

ABSTRACT

The mammalian testis has a special immune microenvironment essential for spermatogenesis. The testis is a remarkable immunoprivileged tissue that protects male germ cells from detrimental immune responses. Various immune cells reside in the testis and are able to regulate spermatogenesis. Numerous immunoregulatory cytokines are produced by testicular cells, and they participate in the regulation of testicular immunoprivileged environment. To overcome the immunoprivileged status and enable effective local defense against microbial infections, most testicular cells adopt the innate immune functions. Therefore, a density of local immunoregulatory networks

[*] Correspondence should be addressed: Daishu Han, PhD; Department of Cell Biology, PUMC & CAMS, 5 Dong Dan San Tiao, Beijing 100005, P. R. China, TEL: 86-10-69156457, Fax: 86-10-69156466, E-mail: dshan@ibms.pumc.edu.cn.

interplay in maintaining testicular immune homeostasis. Disruption of the testicular immune homeostasis may result in orchitis, leading to male infertility. In this article, a review of the current literature on testicular immunoregulation and its underlying mechanisms, along with its effect on testicular functions, is provided.

Keywords: testis, immune privilege, innate immune response, pattern recognition receptor, orchitis; infertility

INTRODUCTION

Mammalian spermatogenesis is a highly organized germ cell differentiation process occurring in the testis. Testosterone synthesis by Leydig cells is another key function of the testis. Testosterone is critical for spermatogenesis, and also regulates the function of various extratesticular target tissues. The testis has a special microenvironment that is essential for its functions. With regard to the immunological aspects, the testis adopts an immunoprivileged environment to protect germ cells from immune attacks [1]. The process of spermatogenesis is completed after puberty, a long time after the establishment of systemic immune self-tolerance during the fetal and neonatal periods. Therefore, the majority of the male germ cells produce a large number of novel autoantigens that are strangers to the immune system. However, these germ cell antigens in the testis are immunologically tolerated under physiological conditions. The mechanisms underlying the testicular immune privilege have been previously investigated and are discussed in this article.

The testis can be infected by a broad spectrum of microbial pathogens, including viruses, bacteria, fungi, and even parasites via circulating blood and ascending genitourinary tract [2]. To overcome immunoprivileged status, the testis adopts an effective local defense system against microorganisms [3]. Various immune cells reside in the testis, and participate in the testicular defense against microbial infections [4]. Testicular cells produce a large panel of cytokines to regulate testicular immune environment [5]. Furthermore, most testicular cells are equipped with the innate immune machinery. Testicular innate immune defense system is also described in this chapter.

Testicular immune homeostasis can be disrupted by microbial infections and autoimmune response, thereby resulting in orchitis and impaired male fertility [6]. Infection of the testis by bacteria, such as *Neisseria gonorrhoeae and Chlamydia trachonatis*, may lead to acute orchitis [7]. Bacterial infections are effectively treated with antibiotics. In contrast, a broad range of viruses may cause chronic orchitis and are associated with male infertility [8]. Autoimmune orchitis is also an etiological factor of male infertility, and pathomechanisms of autoimmune orchitis have been investigated using experimental autoimmune orchitis (EAO) models in rodent animals [9]. Herein, we summarize the immunological disorders in the testis.

1. IMMUNE PRIVILEGE IN THE TESTIS

Mammalian testis is a remarkable immunoprivileged tissue wherein the systemic immune responses to allo- and auto-antigens are significantly reduced. Testicular immune privilege is critical to protect male germ cells from detrimental immune responses. However, the immune privilege can be disrupted under some pathological conditions, thereby leading to autoimmune orchitis and impaired male fertility. Dissection of the mechanisms underlying the testicular immune privilege is essential to develop preventive and therapeutic approaches for orchitis.

1.1. Historical Misconception of Testicular Immune Privilege

Some early studies proposed several misconceptions regarding testicular immune privilege, which need to be clarified. The mammalian testis is anatomically distant from the main body, and the scrotal temperature is ~5 °C below the core body temperature in humans. The low temperature was speculated to contribute to the immunoprivileged status in the testis because immune responses are significantly reduced in cold-blooded vertebrates [10]. It has been reported that the parathyroid allografts in cryptorchid testes and renal subcapsular space survive longer than those placed subcutaneously in the ear, suggesting that the temperature is not a critical factor in testicular immune privilege [11].

Another misconception regarding testicular immune privilege is that the testis has deficient lymphatic drainage. However, an afferent lymphatic vessel between testis and kidney lymph node has been discovered [12]. In fact, most types of immune cells reside in the interstitial spaces of the testis under physiological conditions [13, 14]. Therefore, the sequestration of advanced germ cell antigens from the interstitial immune cells by the blood-testis barrier

(BTB) may contribute to testicular immune privilege. The BTB is formed by adjacent Sertoli cells near the basal lamina, which divides the seminiferous epithelium into adluminal and basal compartments [15]. Notably, early stages of germ cells, including spermatogonia and preleptotene spermatocytes, are located in the basal compartments outside the BTB, and express immunogenic antigens [16]. Allografts in the interstitial spaces enjoy prolonged survival [17]. These observations suggest that the testicular interstitial spaces outside the BTB also possess an immunoprivileged environment. This implies that the BTB is not fully responsible for the immunoprivileged status in the testis. Taken together, the physical structure of the testis is not critical for the maintenance of the immunoprivileged status, and other mechanisms may be involved in the regulation of testicular immune privilege. Substantial evidence suggests that testicular immunoprivileged environment is composed of local immunosuppressive milieu, negative immunoregulatory system, and systemic immune tolerance.

1.2. Local Immunosuppressive Milieu within the Testis

The testicular cells produce numerous immunoregulatory molecules. Several endocrine and paracrine networks comprise an immunosuppressive environment in favor of the immune privilege. Leydig cells synthesize testosterone, and the testosterone plays a crucial role in regulating spermatogenesis. Notably, the testosterone level is 10-fold higher in the testis than in circulation, which is excessive for maintaining normal spermatogenesis. Inhibitory effect of testosterone on the immune responses was proposed because of differences in the immunity between sexes [18]. Testosterone administration has been found to suppress autoimmune diseases in women [19]. Reduction in the levels of testosterone in the testis leads to rapid rejection of intratesticular allografts, suggesting that testosterone inhibits the immune responses and contributes to immune privilege [11]. A recent study showed that testosterone administration inhibits EAO induction in rats [20]. However, testosterone cannot directly act on immune cells, as these cells do not express androgen receptor (AR). In the testis, testosterone targets Sertoli cells that express AR, and indirectly regulate spermatogenesis. Testosterone may therefore regulate testicular immune status by acting on Sertoli cells. Two previous studies have demonstrated that testosterone regulates the permeability of the BTB, and conditional knockout of AR in mouse Sertoli cells results in the disruption of testicular immunoprivileged status [21, 22]. Since the BTB is not fully responsible for testicular immune privilege, it is possible that testosterone participates in immune privilege by regulating the secretion of immunoregulatory cytokines by Sertoli cells.

The testis produces several anti-inflammatory cytokines that can suppress the immune responses in the testis. Transforming growth factor β (TGF-β) family contains three isoforms and has anti-inflammatory activities. TGF-β1 is predominantly produced by Sertoli and Leydig cells [23]. TGF-β1 inhibits immune responses and favors the survival of islet grafts in the testis [24, 25]. Notably, TGF-β receptors are ubiquitously distributed in somatic and germ cells of the testis, suggesting that TGF-β can regulate testicular cell functions [26, 27]. Activin is a homologue of TGF-β, and is known to inhibit inflammation and lymphocyte function [28]. Activin can be secreted by most testicular cells during testis development [29-31]. Activin receptor is expressed in various testicular cells, but predominantly in germ cells [32, 33]. Therefore, activin directly regulates germ cell development [34]. Interleukin-10 (IL-10) is another well-defined anti-inflammatory cytokine in the testis. IL-10 is mainly produced by testicular macrophages [35]. Overexpression of IL-10 in the testis inhibits EAO induction [36].

1.3. Negative Immunoregulatory Systems

Several negative immunoregulatory systems exist in the testis, and contribute to testicular immune privilege by inhibiting the immune responses. The Fas/FasL system is a critical negative immunoregulatory mechanism through the induction of lymphocyte apoptosis [37]. When originally cloned, FasL was found to be highly expressed in the testis [38]. An early study showed that FasL is expressed in Sertoli cells, and plays a critical role in maintaining the immunoprivileged environment of the testis [39]. This conclusion was challenged by a later study, which reported that genetic modification of FasL expression in islet cells failed to protect the islet grafts from immune rejection [40]. Moreover, no correlation was found between FasL expression in Sertoli cells and survival of islets after cotransplantation in non-obese diabetic mice [41]. By contrast, FasL on T cells induced the destruction of islet grafts through the activation of Fas on islet cells [42]. A late study showed that Sertoli cells do not significantly express FasL, whereas male germ cells abundantly express FasL [43]. The function of FasL located on germ cells remains elusive. The programmed death ligand-1/programmed death receptor-1 (PD-L1/PD-1) system also induces T cell apoptosis [44]. PD-

L1 is expressed in male germ cells and plays a role in prolonging the survival of islet graft in the testis [45]. These observations suggest that male germ cells might be implicated in the regulation of testicular immune privilege, and is worthy of further investigation.

Tyro3, Axl and Mer (TAM) belong to a family of receptor tyrosine kinases [46]. Two homologous vitamin K-dependent proteins, growth arrest-specific gene 6 (Gas6) and protein S, are common ligands of TAM receptors [47]. TAM receptors reduce autoimmune responses by promoting the clearance of apoptotic cells [48, 49]. The Gas6/TAM system negatively regulates innate immune responses in antigen-presenting cells [50]. A series of studies demonstrated that the Gas6/TAM system plays a critical role in regulating testicular immune privilege [51]. The Gas6/TAM system is abundantly expressed in the mouse testis [52]. Three TAM receptors are expressed in Sertoli cells. Axl and Mer are also expressed in Leydig cells. Gas6 is exclusively expressed in Leydig cells. TAM receptors may be important in the maintenance of testicular functions because TAM triple knockout male mice are infertile due to impaired spermatogenesis [53]. Notably, Gas6 and TAM receptors are not expressed in male germ cells. Therefore, TAM signaling may indirectly affect spermatogenesis by regulating the functions of Sertoli and Leydig cells [54]. In our previous study, we showed that the Gas6/TAM system facilitates phagocytic removal of apoptotic germ cells by Sertoli cells [55]. The removal of apoptotic cells by phagocytes is an important mechanism to prevent autoimmune diseases [56]. A recent study showed that damaged male germ cells release autoantigens to induce endogenous inflammatory responses in Sertoli cells [57]. Moreover, we demonstrated that the Gas6/TAM system negatively regulates the inflammatory responses in Sertoli cells [58]. Accordingly, TAM triple knockout male mice progressively develop autoimmune orchitis [59]. Furthermore, mice lacking Axl and Mer are susceptible to EAO induction, suggesting that Axl and Mer receptors regulate systemic immune tolerance to germ cell antigens [60]. These observations indicate that Gas6/TAM system may regulate testicular immune privilege at multiple levels.

1.4. Peripheral Immune Tolerance to Male Germ Cell Antigens

Although both local immunosuppressive milieu and peripheral immune tolerance are implicated in the testicular immune privilege, most previous studies focused on the local immunosuppressive milieu. EAO models, which can be induced by immunization of rodent animals with germ cell antigens, have been widely used for investigating the pathogenesis of autoimmune orchitis [61]. Notably, the susceptibility to EAO induction is greatly varied, and depends upon the animal strains. This varied susceptibility can be attributable to differences in the systemic immune tolerance to germ cell antigens. However, the mechanisms underlying the systemic immune tolerance to germ cell autoantigens are largely unknown. Two recent studies showed that the regulators of innate immune responses are involved in EAO induction. Using gene knockout mice, we demonstrated that Toll-like receptor (TLR) 2 and TLR4 cooperatively mediate EAO induction [62]. Interestingly, TLR2 plays a crucial role in mediating autoantibody production. Contrarily, both Axl and Mer inhibit EAO induction [60]. These observations suggest that the innate immune signaling pathways and their negative regulatory systems differently regulate the peripheral immune responses to germ cell antigens. The mechanisms underlying the systemic immune tolerance to germ cell antigens merit further investigation. Particularly, identification of specific autoantigens that induce immune responses can aid in the development of novel diagnostic and therapeutic approaches for the autoimmune orchitis.

2. Resident Leukocytes in the Testis

Most types of systemic immune cells can be found in the testis. These cells are exclusively located in the testicular interstitial spaces. Under physiological conditions, the resident leukocytes regulate testicular functions by secreting cytokines in a paracrine manner, and also participate in the inflammatory responses [4]. Testicular macrophages are major leukocytes in the testis. Other types of leukocytes, including lymphocytes, mast cells, neutrophils and dendritic cells, are also observed in the testis. The numbers of leukocytes vary greatly under physiological and inflammatory conditions. Most studies on the functions of testicular immune cells are performed in murine models. The following data was largely obtained from murine animals.

2.1. Macrophages

Testicular macrophages reside in the interstitial spaces, and represent approximately 20% of total interstitial cells and 80% of leukocytes in the rat testis under physiological conditions [63]. These macrophages interact closely with Leydig cells, and regulate its number and endocrine functions [64, 65]. Testicular macrophages also regulate Sertoli cell function and germ cell differentiation by secreting cytokines in a paracrine manner [66]. However, an increased number of macrophages in the testis is associated with male infertility [67]. There are two subsets of testicular macrophages: ED2 macrophages expressing surface antigen CD163 that can be recognized by ED2 antibody, and ED1 macrophages expressing CD68 that can be recognized by ED1 antibody. ED2 macrophages are resident cells in the testis and exhibit immunosuppressive activities by producing anti-inflammatory cytokines, thus favoring immunoprivileged status. ED1 macrophages are newly arrived cells from circulation and display pro-inflammatory phenotypes [63]. The ratio of ED1 and ED2 macrophage subsets is remarkably altered under inflammatory conditions. ED1 macrophage numbers are dramatically increased and persistent in the testis of EAO models [68]. ED1 macrophages secrete TNF-α and IL-6, and these cytokines induce germ cell apoptosis in EAO [69-71]. Testicular acute inflammatory response due to microbial infections results in a temporary influx of ED1 macrophages, which participate in the clearance of invading microbes [72]. The mechanisms underlying the persistent and temporary presence of circulating ED1 macrophages in autoimmune and infectious orchitis remain elusive.

2.2. Lymphocytes

Lymphocytes are another major population of the testicular immune cells and represent approximately 15% of total leukocytes in the rat testis [73]. Notably, only T lymphocytes but not B cells are found in the testis. All major T cell subsets, including effector, regulatory, and natural killer (NK) T cells, can be observed in the testis. Under physiological conditions, both $CD4^+$ and $CD8^+$ effector T cells reside in the testicular interstitial spaces, with the predominance of $CD8^+$ cells. The T cell subsets can be altered in the rat testis undergoing autoimmune orchitis [14]. Temporary increase in $CD4^+$ cells at the onset of EAO suggests that these cells are involved in the induction of EAO. Further studies showed that $CD4^+$ cells producing Th1 and Th17 cytokines are co-effector cells governing EAO onset, whereas Th1 and Th17 $CD8^+$ cells play roles in maintaining chronic inflammation [74]. Minor regulatory T cells (Tregs) can be found in the rat testis, and Treg numbers increase significantly during EAO development [14]. Particularly, $CD4^+CD25^+$ Tregs inhibit the proliferation of effector T cells in response to testicular antigen stimulation and prolong the survival of islet allografts in the testis [75]. These studies suggest that Tregs suppress inflammatory responses in the testis. NK T cells represent a considerable subset of lymphocytes [76]. Although NK T cells modulate autoimmune responses, the role of these cells in the testis under pathophysiological conditions is unknown.

2.3. Mast Cells

Considerable mast cells are distributed in the normal testis, and EAO induction leads to remarkable increase in their number, suggesting that mast cells may be involved in testicular inflammation [77]. An increase in mast cell numbers in the testis is associated with abnormal spermatogenesis in humans [78]. Mast cells secrete tryptase, an enzyme that induces fibroblast proliferation and collagen synthesis via proteinase-activated receptor 2 (PAR2), thereby resulting in the fibrosis and sclerosis of tissues [79]. PAR2 is abundantly expressed in the peritubular myoid cells and macrophages of the testis, and PAR2 activation leads to testicular inflammation in the rats [77]. Increased mast cell numbers are associated with fibrosis in the testicular biopsies of infertile men [80].

2.4. Dendritic Cells (DCs)

DCs are potent antigen-presenting cells that play crucial roles in linking innate and adaptive immunity. DCs induce the activation and differentiation of lymphocytes in response to allo-antigen stimulation. Conversely, DCs inhibit autoimmune reaction by tolerating T cell response to auto-antigens. Only a small number of DCs are found in the normal rat testis, but EAO induction leads to remarkably increased DCs [81]. The testicular DCs possess immature phenotypes in commitment to the immunoprivileged environment under physiological conditions [82]. However, DCs from the testicular draining lymph nodes of EAO induce the proliferation of "naïve" T cells, suggesting that DCs should be involved in chronic autoimmune orchitis [83]. The role of DCs in EAO development is largely unknown. We hypothesize that the continuous DC-mediated autoantigen presentation to lymphocytes progressively amplifies the autoimmune response, thereby favoring EAO development. Interestingly, Hsp70 is abundantly expressed in male germ cells and functions as an immunodominant autoantigen in rat autoimmune orchitis

[84]. Hsp70 presentation by DCs converts T cell tolerance to autoimmunity, which is in line with our hypothesis [85]. The pathophysiological role of DCs in the testis is worthy of further investigation.

3. Immune Cytokines

Numerous immune cytokines are involved in the regulation of testicular immune responses. These cytokines play both protective and pathogenic roles in the testis. Some of these cytokines directly regulate spermatogenesis and testosterone synthesis under physiological conditions. Several anti-inflammatory cytokines play roles in the maintenance of testicular immune privilege. In contrast, some pro-inflammatory cytokines impair the testicular functions under inflammatory conditions [86, 87]. The roles of major pro-inflammatory cytokines and chemokines in the regulation of testicular functions have been well characterized.

3.1. Pro-Inflammatory Cytokines

Testicular cells constitutively express major pro-inflammatory cytokines like IL-1, IL-6, and TNF-α, which play roles in regulating normal spermatogenesis. However, these cytokines can be significantly upregulated in orchitis and perturb spermatogenesis. There are two IL-1 members, IL-1α and IL-1β. IL-1α is predominantly expressed in Sertoli cells and regulates the division of spermatogonia [88, 89]. IL-1α also modulates endocrine function in the testis by inhibiting the activity of aromatase, an enzyme that converts androgens to estrogens in Sertoli cells [90]. This inhibition is essential for the maintenance of normal spermatogenesis because the overexpression of aromatase impairs spermatogenesis and leads to male infertility in mice [91, 92]. IL-1β is not evidently expressed in the normal testis, but is remarkably upregulated in the testis under inflammatory conditions. Inflammatory stimuli significantly induce IL-1β expression in most types of testicular cells, including Leydig cells, Sertoli cells, and macrophages [93, 94]. High levels of IL-1β perturb steroidogenesis in Leydig cells by inhibiting the expression of P450 steroidogenic enzymes [95, 96]. IL-1α induces the production of IL-6 in Sertoli cells in an autocrine manner [97].

IL-6 is a critical inflammatory factor that promotes the proliferation, differentiation, and activation of lymphocytes. Under physiological conditions, basal levels of IL-6 are detected in Leydig cells, Sertoli cells, and testicular macrophages [98-100]. IL-6 induces transferrin production by Sertoli cells, and inhibits DNA synthesis during meiosis [101, 102]. LPS-induced acute systemic inflammation remarkably upregulates IL-6 in the testis [103]. The upregulation of IL-6 can be induced directly by LPS or indirectly by LPS-induced peripheral TNF-α because both LPS and TNF-α induce IL-6 production in Sertoli cells *in vitro* [104, 105]. IL-6 is dramatically upregulated in the testis of EAO, and is predominantly produced by infiltrated macrophages [71]. Increased IL-6 may perturb testicular functions via different mechanisms. IL-6 induces the apoptosis of germ cells expressing IL-6 receptor in EAO [71]. Subcutaneous administration of IL-6 suppresses the levels of testosterone in men [106]. Correspondingly, IL-6 inhibits LH-induced steroidogenesis in the rat ovary [107].

TNF-α is a potent pro-inflammatory cytokine, and functions differently via two receptors TNFR1 and TNFR2 [108]. TNFR1 signaling induces cell apoptosis via its cytoplasmic death domain [109], whereas TNFR2 lacks the death domain and does not induce cell apoptotic pathway. In contrast, TNFR2 signaling facilitates cell survival and induces inflammatory response through the activation of NF-κB and mitogen-activated protein kinases [110]. Under physiological conditions, TNF-α is predominantly expressed in late stages of germ cells, including pachytene spermatocytes and round spermatids [111]. TNF-α is also faintly detected in the cytoplasm of Sertoli cells [112]. The germ cell stage-dependent expression of TNF-α suggests that this cytokine may be involved in spermatogenesis. TNF-α promotes germ cell survival and inhibits germ cell apoptosis by down-regulating FasL expression [113, 114]. Since TNFR1 and TNFR2 are predominantly expressed in testicular somatic cells, including Leydig, Sertoli, and peritubular cells, TNF-α should be involved in spermatogenesis by regulating the functions of these cells. For instance, TNF-α inhibits steroidogenesis in Leydig cells [115, 116]. TNF-α produced by infiltrating macrophages induces germ cell apoptosis in EAO [70]. The association between germ cell apoptosis and increased TNF-α was also observed in LPS-induced acute testicular inflammation in rats [117]. These observations suggest that TNF-α differently regulates germ cell survival under physiological and inflammatory conditions.

3.2. Chemokines

Chemokines belong to a large family of chemotactic cytokines that guide the migration of immune cells into the infected sites, which are critical for host defense against microbial infections [118]. Chemokines function by binding to their respective receptors, and are grouped into four subfamilies based on the arrangement of the two N-terminal cysteine residues (C) — CXC, CC, XC, and CX3C. These four groups are usually termed as CXC ligand (CXCL), CCL, XCL and CX3CL, and their corresponding receptors as CXCR, CCR, XCR, and CX3CR, respectively.

Testicular roles of the chemokines have yet to be intensively studied because most of them are expressed at very low levels under normal conditions. CCL3 (also termed as MIP-1α) is detected in the testis and regulates germ cell DNA synthesis during spermatogenesis [119]. The expression and regulation of CXCL10 in Leydig cells have been investigated [120]. An alternative CX3CL transcript is found in testicular cells and can be regulated by pro-inflammatory cytokines [121]. Although the chemokines are faintly expressed in the testis under physiological conditions, some of them are remarkably upregulated in the inflamed testis, suggesting that they are involved in testicular inflammatory responses. CCL2 (also termed as MCP-1) is well defined in the testis. The low levels of MCP-1 are detected at in normal rat testis, whereas local injection of LPS leads to significantly upregulated MCP-1 [122]. MCP-1 is predominantly expressed in testicular somatic cells but not in germ cells [123]. Increased expression of MCP-1 is observed in the testis of EAO, suggesting that it participates in the pathogenesis of EAO [124]. CXCL10 expression is dramatically upregulated in testicular cells after being challenged with Sendai virus [125]. Notably, CXCL10 is associated with the pathogenesis of various infectious and autoimmune diseases [126, 127]. The potential role of CXCL10 in the pathogenesis of Sendai virus-induced orchitis remains to be clarified.

4. Innate Immune Responses in Testicular Cells

Although testis is a remarkable immunoprivileged tissue, it is not a sterile site. In fact, various microbial pathogens may infect the testis. To overcome the immune privilege and mount an effective response against invading microbes, the testis constitutes the local innate defense line. In addition to testicular immune cells, which are believed to participate in the testicular defense against microbial infections, recent studies have demonstrated that tissue-specific cells, including Leydig, Sertoli and germ cells, are also equipped with the innate immune machinery. Testicular cells express a large panel of pattern recognition receptors (PRRs). PRRs initiate innate immune responses in testicular cells, and may contribute to testicular defense against microbial infections.

4.1. PRR-Initiated Innate Immune Responses

PRRs belong to a large family of receptors that recognize conserved molecular patterns of microbes, termed as pathogen-associated molecular patterns (PAMPs). PRRs initiate innate immune response and subsequently regulate adaptive immunity against microbial infections [128]. Several families of PRRs, including TLRs, retinoic acid-inducible gene I (RIG-I)-like receptors (RLRs), and cytosolic DNA sensors, have been well characterized [129]. Up to date, 13 TLRs have been identified in mammals, and they belong to transmembrane proteins localized on the plasma or endosomal membrane. TLRs recognize a large spectrum of bacterial, viral, parasitic PAMPs. Most of the TLRs initiate myeloid differentiation protein 88 (MyD88)-dependent pathway, except for TLR3 and TLR4. TLR3 initiates innate immune responses using Toll/IL-1R domain-containing adaptor inducing IFN-β (TRIF), whereas TLR4 initiates both MyD88- and TRIF-dependent pathways. The TLR signaling pathways induce the production of pro-inflammatory cytokines and type 1 IFNs through the activation of nuclear factor kappa B (NF-κB) and interferon regulatory factors (IRFs).

RLR family contains two functional members, RIG-I and melanoma differentiation-associated protein 5 (MDA-5). RIG-I and MDA5 recognize viral double-strand RNA (dsRNA) and initiate an innate antiviral response using a common adaptor IFN-β promoter stimulator-1 (IPS-1) [130]. Several cytosolic DNA sensors, including DNA-dependent activator of IFN regulatory factor, IFN-inducible protein 16 (p204 in mouse), and cGMP-AMP synthase, have been recognized. The cytosolic DNA sensors recognize viral and bacterial DNA, thus initiating innate immune responses using an adaptor protein stimulator of IFN gene (STING) [131]. IPS-1- and STING-dependent pathways induce the expression of pro-inflammatory cytokines and type 1 IFNs through the activation of NF-κB and IRF3. Type 1 IFNs, including IFN-α and IFN-β, induce the production of numerous antiviral proteins, such as

IFN-stimulating gene 15 (ISG15), 2′, 5′-oligoadenylate synthetase (OAS1), and myxovirus resistance 1 (Mx1). These antiviral proteins inhibit viral replication, through different mechanisms [132].

4.2. TLRs in Testicular Cells

Testicular role of TLRs has been recently revealed [131]. TLR signaling has been identified in different murine testicular cells. Several TLRs are expressed in mouse Sertoli cells and initiate innate immune responses after being challenged with their respective ligands [133, 134]. The activation of TLRs in Sertoli cells induce the production of pro-inflammatory cytokines and type 1 IFNs. These findings suggest that Sertoli cells may be involved in testicular innate defense against microbial infections.

Leydig cells are major interstitial cells that synthesize androgens. Leydig cells may be involved in testicular immunoregulation via modulation of the macrophage numbers [135]. Early studies showed that Leydig cells possess innate antiviral properties, and produce IFNs and antiviral proteins in response to viral infection [136, 137]. Recent studies demonstrated that mouse Leydig cells constitutively express TLR3 and TLR4, which can be activated by respective ligands, and induce the expression of pro-inflammatory cytokines and type 1 IFNs through TLR signaling [138]. TLR activation in Leydig cells inhibits androgen synthesis, suggesting that the innate immune responses may perturb testicular functions. Notably, TLR signaling in Sertoli and Leydig cells is negatively regulated by TAM receptors, which would prevent prolonged inflammatory response, thereby impairing testicular functions [58, 138].

Germ cells represent a majority of testicular cells during adulthood, and encounter microbial pathogens from the circulating blood and the ascending genital tract. The innate immune responses to microorganisms in male germ cells should be important in the testicular defense against microbial infections. TLR3 and TLR11 are expressed in mouse male germ cells. TLR3 is predominantly expressed in spermatogonia and spermatocytes [139]. TLR3 signaling induces the expression of pro-inflammatory cytokines and type 1 IFNs in the male germ cells through the activation of NF-κB and IRF3. Moreover, TLR3 activation also induces the expression of antiviral proteins ISG15, OAS1, and Mx1 [139]. TLR3-initiated antiviral response should contribute to the testicular defense against viral infection from the circulating blood and ascending genital tract because spermatogonia and spermatocytes are located in the basal and adluminal compartments of the seminiferous tubules. TLR11 recognizes PAMPs of *T. gondii* and uropathogenic *E. coli* (UPEC), thus initiating innate immune responses against *T. gondii* and UPEC infections in mice [140, 141]. *T. gondii* and UPEC can infect the testis from the ascending genital tract and impair male fertility [142, 143]. TLR11 is abundantly expressed in mouse spermatids and induces the production of IL-12 and IFN-γ after stimulation with *T. gondii* profilin [144]. UPEC infection predominantly induces the production of pro-inflammatory cytokines, including TNF-α, IL-6 and IL-1β, by germ cells through TLR11 signaling. Therefore, spermatids may participate in the testicular defense against *T. gondii* and UPEC infections in mice. However, functional TLR11 is absent in humans [145], which may be a reason why natural *T. gondii* and UPEC infections lead to pathogenesisi in humans, but not in mice.

4.3. RLR-Initiated Antiviral Response in the Testis

The RLR family contains two functional members RIG-I and MDA5, which recognize dsRNA produced during viral replication. RIG-I and MDA5 can also be activated by synthetic dsRNA analog, polyinosinic-polycytidylic acid (poly(I:C)), and initiate innate antiviral response [130]. RIG-I and MDA5 are expressed in Leydig cells, and MDA5 is also detected in spermatids [146]. Poly(I:C) triggers innate antiviral response in Leydig cells and spermatids through IPS-1-dependent pathway, and is characterized by inducing the production of type 1 IFNs and antiviral proteins. Moreover, RIG-I and MDA5 signaling also induces TNF-α and IL-6 production and inhibits testosterone synthesis in Leydig cells, indicating that RLR-mediated innate immune response perturbs testicular functions [146].

4.4. Cytosolic DNA Sensors in Leydig Cells

We recently showed that a cytosolic DNA sensor p204 is abundantly expressed in mouse Leydig cells [147]. Herpes simplex virus DNA analog (HSV60), a synthetic p204 ligand, induces the expression of type 1 IFNs and antiviral proteins through STING-dependent pathway. Notably, p204 signaling in Leydig cells does not inhibit testosterone synthesis, suggesting that DNA sensor signaling may be an ideal strategy for testicular defense against viral infections without the impairment of testicular functions. Testicular antiviral response is interesting because numerous viruses may infect the testis and perturb testicular functions in humans [8]. Notably, human Leydig cells exhibit relatively weak antiviral activities compared with their murine counterparts [148]. Interestingly, natural viral impairment of male fertility is not observed in murines. Delineating the differences in the mechanisms underlying the testicular antiviral system in humans and murine may provide novel clues for the preventive and therapeutic strategies in infertility due to viral infection.

5. Orchitis

The immune privilege and innate immunity in the testis comprise testicular immune homeostasis. Some stimuli, such as microbial infections, chemical toxins, and physical trauma, may disrupt the immune homeostasis in the testis and lead to infectious and autoimmune orchitis, thereby perturbing male fertility [6]. Understanding the pathomechanisms of orchitis can aid in the development of effective treatment approaches.

5.1. Infectious Orchitis

Microbial infections may induce orchitis and perturb testicular functions. *Neisseria gonorrhoeae* and *Chlamydia trachomatis*, the most common sexually transmitted bacteria, predominantly induce acute epididymo-orchitis in young men, whereas *E. coli* commonly infect the genital tract in aged men [149]. Bacterial infections remarkably induce immune cell infiltration and pro-inflammatory cytokine production in the testis of rat models, and compromise testicular functions [117]. Antibiotic treatment is usually effective for bacterial infections.

Viral infection also induces orchitis. Mumps virus has a great testis tropism and may lead to male infertility [150]. Moreover, HIV, coxsackie virus, influenza and dengue viral infections may also result in orchitis [8]. Some other viruses may impair male fertility without orchitis induction [151]. The mechanisms underlying virus-induced orchitis need to be clarified.

5.2. Autoimmune Orchitis

Autoimmune orchitis is a chronic inflammation in the testis, which may result in male infertility. The pathology of autoimmune orchitis has been intensively investigated using EAO models [152]. The activation of $CD4^+$ T cells is critical in the onset of EAO [153]. Persistent macrophage infiltration in the testis is a hallmark of EAO. The infiltrated macrophages produce high levels of pro-inflammatory cytokines such as TNF-α and IL-6, thus inducing germ cell apoptosis [70, 71]. Recent studies showed that $CD4^+$ and $CD8^+$ T cells producing Th1 and Th17 cytokines are involved in the onset of autoimmune orchitis [74]. Although autoimmune orchitis is rare in humans, autoimmune response to sperm results in approximately 7% of male infertile incidences [154].

CONCLUSION

The testis has a special immune environment because of its immunoprivileged status and innate immunity. Disruption of testicular immune homeostasis impairs spermatogenesis and male fertility. Understanding the mechanisms underlying testicular immune environment may provide novel clues for the development of preventive and therapeutic approaches for immunological infertility. Immunobiology of the testis is a broad field. Particularly, the local innate immune defense system against microbial infections in the testis is an important topic for further investigation.

ACKNOWLEDGMENTS

This work was supported by the National Natural Science Foundation of China (Grant Nos. 31171445, 31261160491, 31371518) and the Major State Basic Research Project of China (No. 2015CB943001).

REFERENCES

[1] Li N, Wang T, Han D. Structural, cellular and molecular aspects of immune privilege in the testis. *Front Immunol.* 2012; 3:152.

[2] Bachir BG, Jarvi K. Infectious, inflammatory, and immunologic conditions resulting in male infertility. *Urol Clin North Am.* 2014; 41:67-81.
[3] Zhao S, Zhu W, Xue S, Han D. Testicular defense systems: immune privilege and innate immunity. *Cell Mol Immunol.* 2014; 11:428-437.
[4] Perez CV, Theas MS, Jacobo PV, Jarazo-Dietrich S, Guazzone VA, Lustig L. Dual role of immune cells in the testis: Protective or pathogenic for germ cells? *Spermatogenesis.* 2013; 3:e23870.
[5] Hedger MP, Meinhardt A. Cytokines and the immune-testicular axis. *J Reprod Immunol.* 2003; 58:1-26.
[6] Schuppe HC, Meinhardt A, Allam JP, Bergmann M, Weidner W, Haidl G. Chronic orchitis: a neglected cause of male infertility? *Andrologia.* 2008; 40:84-91.
[7] Ludwig M. Diagnosis and therapy of acute prostatitis, epididymitis and orchitis. *Andrologia.* 2008; 40:76-80.
[8] Dejucq N, Jegou B. Viruses in the mammalian male genital tract and their effects on the reproductive system. *Microbiol Mol Biol Rev.* 2001; 65:208-231.
[9] Jacobo P, Guazzone VA, Theas MS, Lustig L. Testicular autoimmunity. *Autoimmun Rev.* 2011; 10:201-204.
[10] Cone RE, Marchalonis JJ. Cellular and humoral aspects of the influence of environmental temperature on the immune response of poikilothermic vertebrates. *J Immunol.* 1972; 108:952-957.
[11] Head JR, Billingham RE. Immune privilege in the testis. II. Evaluation of potential local factors. *Transplantation.* 1985; 40:269-275.
[12] Head JR, Neaves WB, Billingham RE. Reconsideration of the lymphatic drainage of the rat testis. *Transplantation.* 1983; 35:91-95.
[13] Hedger MP. Testicular leukocytes: what are they doing? *Rev Reprod.* 1997; 2:38-47.
[14] Jacobo P, Guazzone VA, Jarazo-Dietrich S, Theas MS, Lustig L. Differential changes in CD4+ and CD8+ effector and regulatory T lymphocyte subsets in the testis of rats undergoing autoimmune orchitis. *J Reprod Immunol.* 2009; 81:44-54.
[15] Cheng CY, Mruk DD. The blood-testis barrier and its implications for male contraception. *Pharmacol Rev.* 2012; 64:16-64.
[16] Yule TD, Montoya GD, Russell LD, Williams TM, Tung KS. Autoantigenic germ cells exist outside the blood testis barrier. *J Immunol.* 1988; 141:1161-1167.
[17] Immune privilege in the testis. *J Reprod Immunol.* 1990; 18:1-121.

[18] Cutolo M, Sulli A, Capellino S, Villaggio B, Montagna P, Seriolo B, Straub RH. Sex hormones influence on the immune system: basic and clinical aspects in autoimmunity. *Lupus.* 2004; 13:635-638.
[19] Cutolo M. Androgens in rheumatoid arthritis: when are they effectors? *Arthritis Res Ther.* 2009; 11:126.
[20] Fijak M, Schneider E, Klug J, Bhushan S, Hackstein H, Schuler G, Wygrecka M, Gromoll J, Meinhardt A. Testosterone replacement effectively inhibits the development of experimental autoimmune orchitis in rats: evidence for a direct role of testosterone on regulatory T cell expansion. *J Immunol.* 2011; 186:5162-5172.
[21] Meng J, Holdcraft RW, Shima JE, Griswold MD, Braun RE. Androgens regulate the permeability of the blood-testis barrier. *Proc Natl Acad Sci U S A.* 2005; 102:16696-16700.
[22] Meng J, Greenlee AR, Taub CJ, Braun RE. Sertoli cell-specific deletion of the androgen receptor compromises testicular immune privilege in mice. *Biol Reprod.* 2011; 85:254-260.
[23] Avallet O, Vigier M, Leduque P, Dubois PM, Saez JM. Expression and regulation of transforming growth factor-beta 1 messenger ribonucleic acid and protein in cultured porcine Leydig and Sertoli cells. *Endocrinology.* 1994; 134:2079-2087.
[24] Pollanen P, von Euler M, Jahnukainen K, Saari T, Parvinen M, Sainio-Pollanen S, Soder O. Role of transforming growth factor beta in testicular immunosuppression. *J Reprod Immunol.* 1993; 24:123-137.
[25] Suarez-Pinzon W, Korbutt GS, Power R, Hooton J, Rajotte RV, Rabinovitch A. Testicular sertoli cells protect islet beta-cells from autoimmune destruction in NOD mice by a transforming growth factor-beta1-dependent mechanism. *Diabetes.* 2000; 49:1810-1818.
[26] Caussanel V, Tabone E, Hendrick JC, Dacheux F, Benahmed M. Cellular distribution of transforming growth factor betas 1, 2, and 3 and their types I and II receptors during postnatal development and spermatogenesis in the boar testis. *Biol Reprod.* 1997; 56:357-367.
[27] Konrad L, Albrecht M, Renneberg H, Aumuller G. Transforming growth factor-beta2 mediates mesenchymal-epithelial interactions of testicular somatic cells. *Endocrinology.* 2000; 141:3679-3686.
[28] de Kretser DM, Hedger MP, Phillips DJ. Activin A and follistatin: their role in the acute phase reaction and inflammation. *J Endocrinol.* 1999; 161:195-198.
[29] Lee W, Mason AJ, Schwall R, Szonyi E, Mather JP. Secretion of activin by interstitial cells in the testis. *Science.* 1989; 243:396-398.

[30] de Winter JP, Vanderstichele HM, Timmerman MA, Blok LJ, Themmen AP, de Jong FH. Activin is produced by rat Sertoli cells in vitro and can act as an autocrine regulator of Sertoli cell function. *Endocrinology*. 1993; 132:975-982.

[31] de Winter JP, Vanderstichele HM, Verhoeven G, Timmerman MA, Wesseling JG, de Jong FH. Peritubular myoid cells from immature rat testes secrete activin-A and express activin receptor type II in vitro. *Endocrinology*. 1994; 135:759-767.

[32] de Winter JP, Themmen AP, Hoogerbrugge JW, Klaij IA, Grootegoed JA, de Jong FH. Activin receptor mRNA expression in rat testicular cell types. *Mol Cell Endocrinol*. 1992; 83:R1-8.

[33] Kaipia A, Parvinen M, Toppari J. Localization of activin receptor (ActR-IIB2) mRNA in the rat seminiferous epithelium. *Endocrinology*. 1993; 132:477-479.

[34] Meinhardt A, McFarlane JR, Seitz J, de Kretser DM. Activin maintains the condensed type of mitochondria in germ cells. *Mol Cell Endocrinol*. 2000; 168:111-117.

[35] Winnall WR, Muir JA, Hedger MP. Rat resident testicular macrophages have an alternatively activated phenotype and constitutively produce interleukin-10 in vitro. *J Leukoc Biol*. 2011; 90:133-143.

[36] Watanabe M, Kashiwakura Y, Kusumi N, Tamayose K, Nasu Y, Nagai A, Shimada T, Daida H, Kumon H. Adeno-associated virus-mediated human IL-10 gene transfer suppresses the development of experimental autoimmune orchitis. *Gene Ther*. 2005; 12:1126-1132.

[37] Ju ST, Panka DJ, Cui H, Ettinger R, el-Khatib M, Sherr DH, Stanger BZ, Marshak-Rothstein A. Fas (CD95)/FasL interactions required for programmed cell death after T-cell activation. *Nature*. 1995; 373:444-448.

[38] Suda T, Takahashi T, Golstein P, Nagata S. Molecular cloning and expression of the Fas ligand, a novel member of the tumor necrosis factor family. *Cell*. 1993; 75:1169-1178.

[39] Bellgrau D, Gold D, Selawry H, Moore J, Franzusoff A, Duke RC. A role for CD95 ligand in preventing graft rejection. *Nature*. 1995; 377:630-632.

[40] Allison J, Georgiou HM, Strasser A, Vaux DL. Transgenic expression of CD95 ligand on islet beta cells induces a granulocytic infiltration but does not confer immune privilege upon islet allografts. *Proc Natl Acad Sci U S A*. 1997; 94:3943-3947.

[41] Korbutt GS, Suarez-Pinzon WL, Power RF, Rajotte RV, Rabinovitch A.

Testicular Sertoli cells exert both protective and destructive effects on syngeneic islet grafts in non-obese diabetic mice. *Diabetologia.* 2000; 43:474-480.

[42] Suarez-Pinzon WL, Power RF, Rabinovitch A. Fas ligand-mediated mechanisms are involved in autoimmune destruction of islet beta cells in non-obese diabetic mice. *Diabetologia.* 2000; 43:1149-1156.

[43] D'Alessio A, Riccioli A, Lauretti P, Padula F, Muciaccia B, De Cesaris P, Filippini A, Nagata S, Ziparo E. Testicular FasL is expressed by sperm cells. *Proc Natl Acad Sci U S A.* 2001; 98:3316-3321.

[44] Keir ME, Butte MJ, Freeman GJ, Sharpe AH. PD-1 and its ligands in tolerance and immunity. *Annu Rev Immunol.* 2008; 26:677-704.

[45] Cheng X, Dai H, Wan N, Moore Y, Vankayalapati R, Dai Z. Interaction of programmed death-1 and programmed death-1 ligand-1 contributes to testicular immune privilege. *Transplantation.* 2009; 87:1778-1786.

[46] Hafizi S, Dahlback B. Signalling and functional diversity within the Axl subfamily of receptor tyrosine kinases. *Cytokine Growth Factor Rev.* 2006; 17:295-304.

[47] Hafizi S, Dahlback B. Gas6 and protein S. Vitamin K-dependent ligands for the Axl receptor tyrosine kinase subfamily. *FEBS J.* 2006; 273:5231-5244.

[48] Rothlin CV, Lemke G. TAM receptor signaling and autoimmune disease. *Curr Opin Immunol.* 2010; 22:740-746.

[49] Lemke G, Burstyn-Cohen T. TAM receptors and the clearance of apoptotic cells. *Ann N Y Acad Sci.* 2010; 1209:23-29.

[50] Rothlin CV, Ghosh S, Zuniga EI, Oldstone MB, Lemke G. TAM receptors are pleiotropic inhibitors of the innate immune response. *Cell.* 2007; 131:1124-1136.

[51] Deng T, Chen Q, Han D. The roles of TAM receptor tyrosine kinases in the mammalian testis and immunoprivileged sites. *Front Biosci, Landmark.* 2016; 21:316-327.

[52] Wang H, Chen Y, Ge Y, Ma P, Ma Q, Ma J, Wang H, Xue S, Han D. Immunoexpression of Tyro 3 family receptors--Tyro 3, Axl, and Mer--and their ligand Gas6 in postnatal developing mouse testis. *J Histochem Cytochem.* 2005; 53:1355-1364.

[53] Lu Q, Gore M, Zhang Q, Camenisch T, Boast S, Casagranda F, Lai C, Skinner MK, Klein R, Matsushima GK, Earp HS, Goff SP, Lemke G. Tyro-3 family receptors are essential regulators of mammalian spermatogenesis. *Nature.* 1999; 398:723-728.

[54] Chen Y, Wang H, Qi N, Wu H, Xiong W, Ma J, Lu Q, Han D.

Functions of TAM RTKs in regulating spermatogenesis and male fertility in mice. *Reproduction.* 2009; 138:655-666.

[55] Xiong W, Chen Y, Wang H, Wang H, Wu H, Lu Q, Han D. Gas6 and the Tyro 3 receptor tyrosine kinase subfamily regulate the phagocytic function of Sertoli cells. *Reproduction.* 2008; 135:77-87.

[56] Nagata S, Hanayama R, Kawane K. Autoimmunity and the clearance of dead cells. *Cell.* 2010; 140:619-630.

[57] Zhang X, Wang T, Deng T, Xiong W, Lui P, Li N, Chen Y, Han D. Damaged spermatogenic cells induce inflammatory gene expression in mouse Sertoli cells through the activation of Toll-like receptors 2 and 4. *Mol Cell Endocrinol.* 2013; 365:162-173.

[58] Sun B, Qi N, Shang T, Wu H, Deng T, Han D. Sertoli cell-initiated testicular innate immune response through toll-like receptor-3 activation is negatively regulated by Tyro3, Axl, and mer receptors. *Endocrinology.* 2010; 151:2886-2897.

[59] Zhang Y, Li N, Chen Q, Yan K, Liu Z, Zhang X, Liu P, Chen Y, Han D. Breakdown of immune homeostasis in the testis of mice lacking Tyro3, Axl and Mer receptor tyrosine kinases. *Immunol Cell Biol.* 2013; 91:416-426.

[60] Li N, Liu Z, Zhang Y, Chen Q, Liu P, Cheng CY, Lee WM, Chen Y, Han D. Mice lacking Axl and Mer tyrosine kinase receptors are susceptible to experimental autoimmune orchitis induction. *Immunol Cell Biol.* 2015; 93:311-320.

[61] Naito M, Terayama H, Hirai S, Qu N, Lustig L, Itoh M. Experimental autoimmune orchitis as a model of immunological male infertility. *Med Mol Morphol.* 2012; 45:185-189.

[62] Liu Z, Zhao S, Chen Q, Yan K, Liu P, Li N, Cheng CY, Lee WM, Han D. Roles of Toll-like receptors 2 and 4 in mediating experimental autoimmune orchitis induction in mice. *Biol Reprod.* 2015; 92:63.

[63] Hedger MP. Macrophages and the immune responsiveness of the testis. *J Reprod Immunol.* 2002; 57:19-34.

[64] Hutson JC. Physiologic interactions between macrophages and Leydig cells. *Exp Biol Med.* 2006; 231:1-7.

[65] Gaytan F, Bellido C, Aguilar E, van Rooijen N. Requirement for testicular macrophages in Leydig cell proliferation and differentiation during prepubertal development in rats. *J Reprod Fertil.* 1994; 102:393-399.

[66] Cohen PE, Nishimura K, Zhu L, Pollard JW. Macrophages: important accessory cells for reproductive function. *J Leukoc Biol.* 1999;

66(5):765-772.

[67] Frungieri MB, Calandra RS, Lustig L, Meineke V, Kohn FM, Vogt HJ, Mayerhofer A. Number, distribution pattern, and identification of macrophages in the testes of infertile men. *Fertil Steril.* 2002; 78:298-306.

[68] Rival C, Theas MS, Suescun MO, Jacobo P, Guazzone V, van Rooijen N, Lustig L. Functional and phenotypic characteristics of testicular macrophages in experimental autoimmune orchitis. *J Pathol.* 2008; 215:108-117.

[69] Suescun MO, Rival C, Theas MS, Calandra RS, Lustig L. Involvement of tumor necrosis factor-alpha in the pathogenesis of autoimmune orchitis in rats. *Biol Reprod.* 2003; 68:2114-2121.

[70] Theas MS, Rival C, Jarazo-Dietrich S, Jacobo P, Guazzone VA, Lustig L. Tumour necrosis factor-alpha released by testicular macrophages induces apoptosis of germ cells in autoimmune orchitis. *Hum Reprod.* 2008; 23:1865-1872.

[71] Rival C, Theas MS, Guazzone VA, Lustig L. Interleukin-6 and IL-6 receptor cell expression in testis of rats with autoimmune orchitis. *J Reprod Immunol.* 2006; 70:43-58.

[72] Gerdprasert O, O'Bryan MK, Muir JA, Caldwell AM, Schlatt S, de Kretser DM, Hedger MP. The response of testicular leukocytes to lipopolysaccharide-induced inflammation: further evidence for heterogeneity of the testicular macrophage population. *Cell Tissue Res.* 2002; 308:277-285.

[73] Hedger MP, Meinhardt A. Local regulation of T cell numbers and lymphocyte-inhibiting activity in the interstitial tissue of the adult rat testis. *J Reprod Immunol.* 2000; 48:69-80.

[74] Jacobo P, Perez CV, Theas MS, Guazzone VA, Lustig L. CD4+ and CD8+ T cells producing Th1 and Th17 cytokines are involved in the pathogenesis of autoimmune orchitis. *Reproduction.* 2011; 141:249-258.

[75] Nasr IW, Wang Y, Gao G, Deng S, Diggs L, Rothstein DM, Tellides G, Lakkis FG, Dai Z. Testicular immune privilege promotes transplantation tolerance by altering the balance between memory and regulatory T cells. *J Immunol.* 2005; 174:6161-6168.

[76] Tompkins AB, Hutchinson P, de Kretser DM, Hedger MP. Characterization of lymphocytes in the adult rat testis by flow cytometry: effects of activin and transforming growth factor beta on lymphocyte subsets in vitro. *Biol Reprod.* 1998; 58:943-951.

[77] Iosub R, Klug J, Fijak M, Schneider E, Frohlich S, Blumbach K, Wennemuth G, Sommerhoff CP, Steinhoff M, Meinhardt A. Development of testicular inflammation in the rat involves activation of proteinase-activated receptor-2. *J Pathol.* 2006; 208:686-698.
[78] Hussein MR, Abou-Deif ES, Bedaiwy MA, Said TM, Mustafa MG, Nada E, Ezat A, Agarwal A. Phenotypic characterization of the immune and mast cell infiltrates in the human testis shows normal and abnormal spermatogenesis. *Fertil Steril.* 2005; 83:1447-1453.
[79] Abe M, Kurosawa M, Ishikawa O, Miyachi Y, Kido H. Mast cell tryptase stimulates both human dermal fibroblast proliferation and type I collagen production. *Clin Exp Allergy.* 1998; 28:1509-1517.
[80] Apa DD, Cayan S, Polat A, Akbay E. Mast cells and fibrosis on testicular biopsies in male infertility. *Arch Androl.* 2002; 48:337-344.
[81] Rival C, Lustig L, Iosub R, Guazzone VA, Schneider E, Meinhardt A, Fijak M. Identification of a dendritic cell population in normal testis and in chronically inflamed testis of rats with autoimmune orchitis. *Cell Tissue Res.* 2006; 324:311-318.
[82] Rival C, Guazzone VA, von Wulffen W, Hackstein H, Schneider E, Lustig L, Meinhardt A, Fijak M. Expression of co-stimulatory molecules, chemokine receptors and proinflammatory cytokines in dendritic cells from normal and chronically inflamed rat testis. *Mol Hum Reprod.* 2007; 13:853-861.
[83] Guazzone VA, Hollwegs S, Mardirosian M, Jacobo P, Hackstein H, Wygrecka M, Schneider E, Meinhardt A, Lustig L, Fijak M. Characterization of dendritic cells in testicular draining lymph nodes in a rat model of experimental autoimmune orchitis. *Int J Androl.* 2011; 34:276-289.
[84] Fijak M, Iosub R, Schneider E, Linder M, Respondek K, Klug J, Meinhardt A. Identification of immunodominant autoantigens in rat autoimmune orchitis. *J Pathol.* 2005; 207:127-138.
[85] Millar DG, Garza KM, Odermatt B, Elford AR, Ono N, Li Z, Ohashi PS. Hsp70 promotes antigen-presenting cell function and converts T-cell tolerance to autoimmunity in vivo. *Nat Med.* 2003; 9:1469-1476.
[86] Bornstein SR, Rutkowski H, Vrezas I. Cytokines and steroidogenesis. *Mol Cell Endocrinol.* 2004; 215:135-141.
[87] Guazzone VA, Jacobo P, Theas MS, Lustig L. Cytokines and chemokines in testicular inflammation: A brief review. *Microsc Res Tech.* 2009; 72:620-628.
[88] Gerard N, Syed V, Bardin W, Genetet N, Jegou B. Sertoli cells are the

site of interleukin-1 alpha synthesis in rat testis. *Mol Cell Endocrinol.* 1991; 82:R13-16.

[89] Soder O, Syed V, Callard GV, Toppari J, Pollanen P, Parvinen M, Froysa B, Ritzen EM. Production and secretion of an interleukin-1-like factor is stage-dependent and correlates with spermatogonial DNA synthesis in the rat seminiferous epithelium. *Int J Andrology.* 1991; 14:223-231.

[90] Khan SA, Nieschlag E. Interleukin-1 inhibits follitropin-induced aromatase activity in immature rat Sertoli cells in vitro. *Mol Cell Endocrinol.* 1991; 75:1-7.

[91] Li X, Nokkala E, Yan W, Streng T, Saarinen N, Warri A, Huhtaniemi I, Santti R, Makela S, Poutanen M. Altered structure and function of reproductive organs in transgenic male mice overexpressing human aromatase. *Endocrinology.* 2001; 142:2435-2442.

[92] Li X, Strauss L, Makela S, Streng T, Huhtaniemi I, Santti R, Poutanen M. Multiple structural and functional abnormalities in the p450 aromatase expressing transgenic male mice are ameliorated by a p450 aromatase inhibitor. *Am J Pathol.* 2004; 164:1039-1048.

[93] Cudicini C, Lejeune H, Gomez E, Bosmans E, Ballet F, Saez J, Jegou B. Human Leydig cells and Sertoli cells are producers of interleukins-1 and -6. *J Clin Endocrinol Metab.* 1997; 82:1426-1433.

[94] Xiong Y, Hales DB. Expression, regulation, and production of tumor necrosis factor-alpha in mouse testicular interstitial macrophages in vitro. *Endocrinology.* 1993; 133:2568-2573.

[95] Lin T, Wang TL, Nagpal ML, Calkins JH, Chang WW, Chi R. Interleukin-1 inhibits cholesterol side-chain cleavage cytochrome P450 expression in primary cultures of Leydig cells. *Endocrinology.* 1991; 129:1305-1311.

[96] Hales DB. Interleukin-1 inhibits Leydig cell steroidogenesis primarily by decreasing 17 alpha-hydroxylase/C17-20 lyase cytochrome P450 expression. *Endocrinology.* 1992; 131:2165-2172.

[97] Syed V, Stephan JP, Gerard N, Legrand A, Parvinen M, Bardin CW, Jegou B. Residual bodies activate Sertoli cell interleukin-1 alpha (IL-1 alpha) release, which triggers IL-6 production by an autocrine mechanism, through the lipoxygenase pathway. *Endocrinology.* 1995; 136:3070-3078.

[98] Cudicini C, Kercret H, Touzalin AM, Ballet F, Jegou B. Vectorial production of interleukin 1 and interleukin 6 by rat Sertoli cells cultured in a dual culture compartment system. *Endocrinology.* 1997; 138:2863-

2870.
[99] Boockfor FR, Wang D, Lin T, Nagpal ML, Spangelo BL. Interleukin-6 secretion from rat Leydig cells in culture. *Endocrinology.* 1994; 134:2150-2155.
[100] Kern S, Robertson SA, Mau VJ, Maddocks S. Cytokine secretion by macrophages in the rat testis. *Biol Reprod.* 1995; 53:1407-1416.
[101] Boockfor FR, Schwarz LK. Effects of interleukin-6, interleukin-2, and tumor necrosis factor alpha on transferrin release from Sertoli cells in culture. *Endocrinology.* 1991; 129:256-262.
[102] Hakovirta H, Syed V, Jegou B, Parvinen M. Function of interleukin-6 as an inhibitor of meiotic DNA synthesis in the rat seminiferous epithelium. *Mol Cell Endocrinol.* 1995; 108:193-198.
[103] Elhija MA, Potashnik H, Lunenfeld E, Potashnik G, Schlatt S, Nieschlag E, Huleihel M. Testicular interleukin-6 response to systemic inflammation. *Eur Cytokine Netw.* 2005; 16:167-172.
[104] Riccioli A, Filippini A, De Cesaris P, Barbacci E, Stefanini M, Starace G, Ziparo E. Inflammatory mediators increase surface expression of integrin ligands, adhesion to lymphocytes, and secretion of interleukin 6 in mouse Sertoli cells. *Proc Natl Acad Sci U S A.* 1995; 92:5808-5812.
[105] Stephan JP, Syed V, Jegou B. Regulation of Sertoli cell IL-1 and IL-6 production in vitro. *Mol Cell Endocrinol.* 1997; 134:109-118.
[106] Tsigos C, Papanicolaou DA, Kyrou I, Raptis SA, Chrousos GP. Dose-dependent effects of recombinant human interleukin-6 on the pituitary-testicular axis. *J Interferon Cytokine Res.* 1999; 19:1271-1276.
[107] Van der Hoek KH, Woodhouse CM, Brannstrom M, Norman RJ. Effects of interleukin (IL)-6 on luteinizing hormone- and IL-1beta-induced ovulation and steroidogenesis in the rat ovary. *Biol Reprod.* 1998; 58:1266-1271.
[108] Dempsey PW, Doyle SE, He JQ, Cheng G. The signaling adaptors and pathways activated by TNF superfamily. *Cytokine Growth Factor Rev.* 2003; 14:193-209.
[109] Chen G, Goeddel DV. TNF-R1 signaling: a beautiful pathway. *Science.* 2002; 296:1634-1635.
[110] Faustman D, Davis M. TNF receptor 2 pathway: drug target for autoimmune diseases. *Nat Rev Drug Discov.* 2010; 9:482-493.
[111] De SK, Chen HL, Pace JL, Hunt JS, Terranova PF, Enders GC. Expression of tumor necrosis factor-alpha in mouse spermatogenic cells. *Endocrinology.* 1993; 133:389-396.
[112] Siu MK, Lee WM, Cheng CY. The interplay of collagen IV, tumor

necrosis factor-alpha, gelatinase B (matrix metalloprotease-9), and tissue inhibitor of metalloproteases-1 in the basal lamina regulates Sertoli cell-tight junction dynamics in the rat testis. *Endocrinology.* 2003; 144:371-387.

[113] Suominen JS, Wang Y, Kaipia A, Toppari J. Tumor necrosis factor-alpha (TNF-alpha) promotes cell survival during spermatogenesis, and this effect can be blocked by infliximab, a TNF-alpha antagonist. *Eur J Endocrinol.* 2004; 151:629-640.

[114] Pentikainen V, Erkkila K, Suomalainen L, Otala M, Pentikainen MO, Parvinen M, Dunkel L. TNFalpha down-regulates the Fas ligand and inhibits germ cell apoptosis in the human testis. *J Clin Endocrinol Metab.* 2001; 86:4480-4488.

[115] Xiong Y, Hales DB. The role of tumor necrosis factor-alpha in the regulation of mouse Leydig cell steroidogenesis. *Endocrinology.* 1993; 132:2438-2444.

[116] Hong CY, Park JH, Ahn RS, Im SY, Choi HS, Soh J, Mellon SH, Lee K. Molecular mechanism of suppression of testicular steroidogenesis by proinflammatory cytokine tumor necrosis factor alpha. *Mol Cell Biol.* 2004; 24:2593-2604.

[117] O'Bryan MK, Schlatt S, Phillips DJ, de Kretser DM, Hedger MP. Bacterial lipopolysaccharide-induced inflammation compromises testicular function at multiple levels in vivo. *Endocrinology.* 2000; 141:238-246.

[118] Sokol CL, Luster AD. The chemokine system in innate immunity. *Cold Spring Harb Perspect Biol.* 2015; 7.

[119] Hakovirta H, Vierula M, Wolpe SD, Parvinen M. MIP-1 alpha is a regulator of mitotic and meiotic DNA synthesis during spermatogenesis. *Mol Cell Endocrinol.* 1994; 99:119-124.

[120] Hu J, You S, Li W, Wang D, Nagpal ML, Mi Y, Liang P, Lin T. Expression and regulation of interferon-gamma-inducible protein 10 gene in rat Leydig cells. *Endocrinology.* 1998; 139:3637-3645.

[121] Habasque C, Satie AP, Aubry F, Jegou B, Samson M. Expression of fractalkine in the rat testis: molecular cloning of a novel alternative transcript of its gene that is differentially regulated by pro-inflammatory cytokines. *Mol Hum Reprod.* 2003; 9:449-455.

[122] Gerdprasert O, O'Bryan MK, Nikolic-Paterson DJ, Sebire K, de Kretser DM, Hedger MP. Expression of monocyte chemoattractant protein-1 and macrophage colony-stimulating factor in normal and inflamed rat testis. *Mol Hum Reprod.* 2002; 8:518-524.

[123] Aubry F, Habasque C, Satie AP, Jegou B, Samson M. Expression and regulation of the CC-chemokine monocyte chemoattractant protein-1 in rat testicular cells in primary culture. *Biol Reprod.* 2000; 62(5):1427-1435.

[124] Guazzone VA, Rival C, Denduchis B, Lustig L. Monocyte chemoattractant protein-1 (MCP-1/CCL2) in experimental autoimmune orchitis. *J Reprod Immunol.* 2003; 60:143-157.

[125] Le Goffic R, Mouchel T, Aubry F, Patard JJ, Ruffault A, Jegou B, Samson M. Production of the chemokines monocyte chemotactic protein-1, regulated on activation normal T cell expressed and secreted protein, growth-related oncogene, and interferon-gamma-inducible protein-10 is induced by the Sendai virus in human and rat testicular cells. *Endocrinology.* 2002; 143:1434-1440.

[126] Liu M, Guo S, Hibbert JM, Jain V, Singh N, Wilson NO, Stiles JK. CXCL10/IP-10 in infectious diseases pathogenesis and potential therapeutic implications. *Cytokine Growth Factor Rev.* 2011; 22:121-130.

[127] Antonelli A, Ferrari SM, Giuggioli D, Ferrannini E, Ferri C, Fallahi P. Chemokine (C-X-C motif) ligand (CXCL)10 in autoimmune diseases. *Autoimmun Rev.* 2014; 13:272-280.

[128] Iwasaki A, Medzhitov R. Control of adaptive immunity by the innate immune system. *Nat Immunol.* 2015; 16:343-353.

[129] Kumar H, Kawai T, Akira S. Pathogen recognition by the innate immune system. *Int Rev Immunol.* 2011; 30:16-34.

[130] Loo YM, Gale M, Jr. Immune signaling by RIG-I-like receptors. *Immunity.* 2011; 34:680-692.

[131] Orzalli MH, Knipe DM. Cellular sensing of viral DNA and viral evasion mechanisms. *Annu Rev Microbiol.* 2014; 68:477-492.

[132] Sadler AJ, Williams BR. Interferon-inducible antiviral effectors. *Nat Rev Immunol.* 2008; 8:559-568.

[133] Riccioli A, Starace D, Galli R, Fuso A, Scarpa S, Palombi F, De Cesaris P, Ziparo E, Filippini A. Sertoli cells initiate testicular innate immune responses through TLR activation. *J Immunol.* 2006; 177:7122-7130.

[134] Wu H, Wang H, Xiong W, Chen S, Tang H, Han D. Expression patterns and functions of toll-like receptors in mouse sertoli cells. *Endocrinology.* 2008; 149:4402-4412.

[135] Raburn DJ, Coquelin A, Reinhart AJ, Hutson JC. Regulation of the macrophage population in postnatal rat testis. *J Reprod Immunol.* 1993; 24:139-151.

[136] Melaine N, Lienard MO, Guillaume E, Ruffault A, Dejucq-Rainsford N, Jegou B. Production of the antiviral proteins 2'5'oligoadenylate synthetase, PKR and Mx in interstitial cells and spermatogonia. *J Reprod Immunol.* 2003; 59:53-60.

[137] Dejucq N, Lienard MO, Guillaume E, Dorval I, Jegou B. Expression of interferons-alpha and -gamma in testicular interstitial tissue and spermatogonia of the rat. *Endocrinology.* 1998; 139:3081-3087.

[138] Shang T, Zhang X, Wang T, Sun B, Deng T, Han D. Toll-like receptor-initiated testicular innate immune responses in mouse Leydig cells. *Endocrinology.* 2011; 152:2827-2836.

[139] Wang T, Zhang X, Chen Q, Deng T, Zhang Y, Li N, Shang T, Chen Y, Han D. Toll-like receptor 3-initiated antiviral responses in mouse male germ cells in vitro. *Biol Reprod.* 2012; 86(4):106.

[140] Zhang D, Zhang G, Hayden MS, Greenblatt MB, Bussey C, Flavell RA, Ghosh S. A toll-like receptor that prevents infection by uropathogenic bacteria. *Science.* 2004; 303:1522-1526.

[141] Yarovinsky F, Zhang D, Andersen JF, Bannenberg GL, Serhan CN, Hayden MS, Hieny S, Sutterwala FS, Flavell RA, Ghosh S, Sher A. TLR11 activation of dendritic cells by a protozoan profilin-like protein. *Science.* 2005; 308:1626-1629.

[142] Terpsidis KI, Papazahariadou MG, Taitzoglou IA, Papaioannou NG, Georgiadis MP, Theodoridis IT. Toxoplasma gondii: reproductive parameters in experimentally infected male rats. *Exp Parasitol.* 2009; 121:238-241.

[143] Lu Y, Bhushan S, Tchatalbachev S, Marconi M, Bergmann M, Weidner W, Chakraborty T, Meinhardt A. Necrosis is the dominant cell death pathway in uropathogenic Escherichia coli elicited epididymo-orchitis and is responsible for damage of rat testis. *PloS One.* 2013; 8:e52919.

[144] Chen Q, Zhu W, Liu Z, Yan K, Zhao S, Han D. Toll-like receptor 11-initiated innate immune response in male mouse germ cells. *Biol Reprod.* 2014; 90:38.

[145] Lauw FN, Caffrey DR, Golenbock DT. Of mice and man: TLR11 (finally) finds profilin. *Trends Immunol.* 2005; 26:509-511.

[146] Zhu W, Chen Q, Yan K, Liu Z, Li N, Zhang X, Yu L, Chen Y, Han D. RIG-I-like receptors mediate innate antiviral response in mouse testis. *Mol Endocrinol.* 2013; 27:1455-1467.

[147] Zhu W, Liu P, Yu L, Chen Q, Liu Z, Yan K, Lee WM, Cheng CY, Han D. p204-initiated innate antiviral response in mouse Leydig cells. *Biol Reprod.* 2014; 91:8.

[148] Le Tortorec A, Denis H, Satie AP, Patard JJ, Ruffault A, Jegou B, Dejucq-Rainsford N. Antiviral responses of human Leydig cells to mumps virus infection or poly I:C stimulation. *Hum Reprod.* 2008; 23:2095-2103.
[149] Trojian TH, Lishnak TS, Heiman D. Epididymitis and orchitis: an overview. *Am Fam Physician.* 2009; 79:583-587.
[150] Masarani M, Wazait H, Dinneen M. Mumps orchitis. *J R Soc Med.* 2006; 99:573-575.
[151] Garolla A, Pizzol D, Bertoldo A, Menegazzo M, Barzon L, Foresta C. Sperm viral infection and male infertility: focus on HBV, HCV, HIV, HPV, HSV, HCMV, and AAV. *J Reprod Immunol.* 2013; 100:20-29.
[152] Rival C, Guazzone VA, Theas MS, Lustig L. Pathomechanism of autoimmune orchitis. *Andrologia.* 2005; 37:226-227.
[153] Mahi-Brown CA, Tung KS. Activation requirements of donor T cells and host T cell recruitment in adoptive transfer of murine experimental autoimmune orchitis (EAO). *Cell Immunol.* 1989; 124:368-379.
[154] Hendry WF. Detection and treatment of antispermatozoal antibodies in men. *Reprod Fertil Dev.* 1989; 1:205-220.

INDEX

A

A spermatogonia, 32, 49, 51
acetylation, 59
acid, 4, 7, 17, 21, 38, 50, 60, 67, 83, 85
acrosome, vii, 1, 2, 3, 4, 5, 6, 7, 8, 9, 10, 11, 12, 13, 14, 16, 17, 18, 19, 20, 21, 22, 23, 24, 25, 26, 27, 29, 32
activating transcription factor 1 (*Atf1*), 38
adaptive immunity, 79, 83, 98
adenylation, 35
adhesion, 12, 96
AGO, 34, 40
anchoring, vii, 1, 10, 11, 12, 27
androgen(s), 74, 80, 84, 89
annotation, 52, 54, 58
antibody, 78
antigen-presenting cell(s), 76, 79, 94
antisense, 35, 39, 41, 43, 47, 48, 57, 61, 68
antisense RNA, 39, 61
APC/C (the anaphase promoting complex/cyclosome), 41, 70
apoptosis, 34, 38, 39, 43, 50, 59, 62, 75, 78, 81, 87, 93, 97
arginine, 55
Argonaute, 36, 37, 66
Argonaute (AGO), 36, 37
Asz1, 46
autoantigens, 72, 76, 77, 94
autoimmune disease(s), 74, 76, 82, 91, 96, 98
autoimmune orchitis, 87
autoimmunity, 80, 88, 89, 94

B

B spermatogonia, 32
bacteria, 72, 86, 99
bacterial infection, 86
basal lamina, 74, 97
base pair, 36, 37
bile, 4, 17
biochemistry, 16
biological processes, 36
biosynthesis, 29, 39
blood-testis barrier (BTB), 73, 74, 88, 89
brain, 69
budding, 6, 7, 19

C

carbohydrate, 16
carboxylesterase 7 (Ces7), 48, 50
carcinoma, 51, 62, 64
casein, 27
catalysis, 65
CCR, 82
CD163, 78
CD8+, 78, 87, 88, 93

CD95, 90
cDNA, 22
cell biology, 18, 19, 20, 22, 23, 24, 25, 52
cell death, 90, 99
cell differentiation, viii, 32, 33, 34, 55, 57, 63, 72, 78
cell fate, 36
cell line, 57
cell surface, 24
chaperones, 17
chemokine receptor, 94
chemokines, 80, 82, 94, 98
chlamydia, 73, 86
chlamydia trachomatis, 86
cholesterol, 50, 95
chromatin, vii, 2, 32, 33, 38, 44, 48, 63
chromatin assembly factor 1 (Caf1), 44
chromatin modifiers, 63
chromatoid body (CB), 33, 46
chromosome, 45, 69
cilium, 25
circular lncRNAs (ciRNAs), 47
circulation, 74, 78
classes, 41, 46, 47
cloning, 22, 90, 97
clusters, 34, 35, 38, 41, 42, 49, 53, 60, 67, 69
coding, 34, 35, 36, 41, 42, 44, 46, 49, 50, 51, 52, 55, 56, 57, 58, 61, 62, 63, 64, 67, 68
colitis, 21
collagen, 79, 94, 96
compaction, 11, 32, 38
complementarity, 44
condensation, vii, 2, 32, 38
conditional knockout (cKO), 4, 39, 74
conservation, 46, 48, 56
culture, 95, 96, 98
CXC, 82
cysteine, 82
cytochrome, 18, 95
cytokines, viii, 71, 72, 75, 77, 78, 80, 82, 83, 84, 87, 93, 94, 97
cytology, 15, 27
cytometry, 93
cytoplasm, 35, 37, 46, 51, 60, 81
cytoskeleton, 5, 13, 24

D

dark matter, 64, 67
database, 35, 47, 65
days postcoitum (dpc), 40
days postpartum (dpp), 40
DEAD (Asp-Glu-Ala-Asp) box polypeptide 4 (Ddx4), 46
decay, 45, 61
defects, 9, 20, 39, 43
deficiency, 10, 20, 22
degradation, 30, 34, 41, 42, 46, 48, 51
dendritic cell (DCs), 77, 79, 94, 99
dengue, 86
destruction, 75, 89, 91
detachment, 11, 12
developing brain, 17
developmental change, 59
diabetes, 89
Dicer, 34, 35, 39, 42
Dicer cKO mice, 39
differentially methylated regions (DMRs), 45
differentiation, vii, viii, 2, 20, 32, 33, 34, 38, 51, 55, 57, 60, 63, 67, 72, 78, 79, 81, 83, 92
DiGeorge syndrome critical region 8 (DGCR8), 35, 37, 39, 58, 70
diplotene, 33
distribution, 89, 93
diversity, 36, 91
Dlx6os1, distal-less homeobox 6, opposite strand 1, 48
Dmrt1-Related Gene (Dmr), 50
DNA, 30, 33, 36, 42, 43, 44, 45, 48, 53, 59, 60, 61, 68, 69, 81, 82, 83, 85, 95, 96, 97, 98
DNA damage, 60
DNA repair, 30
DNA strand breaks, 33
docosahexaenoic acid, 7

doublesex and mab-3 related transcription factor 1 (Dmrt1), 50, 53, 69
double-strands RNAs (dsRNAs), 36, 37
dpc, 33, 40, 45, 49
dpp, 33, 40, 49
drainage, 73, 88
Drosha, 35, 37, 39, 58, 62
Drosha KO mice, 39
drosophila, 15, 25, 39, 56, 58, 60, 64, 65, 68, 70

E

E. coli, 85, 86
E2f1, 38
Eif3A, 45
Eif4E, 45
Eif4G, 45
elongating spermatids, 11, 32, 33, 45
elongation, 26, 44
elucidation, 52
embryogenesis, 65
embryonic stem cells (ESCs), 39, 68
encoding, 23
endocrine, 66, 74, 78, 80
endogenous small-interfering RNAs (endo-siRNAs), vii, viii, 31, 32, 34, 39, 40, 42, 46, 55, 57, 64, 70
endonuclease, 56, 63
Endo-siRNAs Biogenesis, 39
enhancer RNAs (eRNAs), 47
environment, viii, 71, 72, 74, 75, 79, 87
enzyme(s), 2, 8, 13, 16, 18, 23, 69, 79, 80
epididymis, 48, 50
epididymitis, 88
epigenetics, 48, 52, 55
epithelium, 15, 32, 64, 74, 90, 95, 96
eukaryotic, 45, 47, 60
eukaryotic cell, 60
eukaryotic translation initiation factor (Eif), 45
evolution, 57, 61, 67
exons, 10, 41, 42, 47
experimental autoimmune orchitis (EAO), 73, 74, 75, 76, 78, 79, 81, 82, 87, 89, 90, 92, 93, 94, 98, 100
exportin 5 (EXP5), 35

F

fatty acids, 7
fertility, vii, 1, 18, 24, 27, 35, 39, 44, 65, 68, 70, 72, 73, 85, 86, 87, 92
fertilization, 2, 15, 16, 57
fibroblast proliferation, 79, 94
fibrosis, 79, 94
flagellum, vii, 2, 32, 46, 59
formation, viii, 5, 6, 7, 8, 9, 11, 16, 18, 19, 20, 21, 22, 23, 31, 32, 33, 44, 55, 58, 68
fusion, vii, 1, 5, 6, 7, 9, 17, 19, 21, 22

G

gametogenesis, 43
gastrulation, 67
GENCODE, 47, 56, 57, 58
gene expression, viii, 31, 34, 37, 48, 49, 52, 61, 62, 66, 67, 68, 92
gene regulation, 48, 68
gene silencing, 43, 48, 63, 64
gene transfer, 90
genes, 5, 11, 14, 15, 34, 35, 36, 37, 41, 42, 45, 47, 48, 49, 51, 54, 58, 59, 61, 62, 65, 67, 68
genetics, 28
genitourinary tract, 72
genome, viii, 14, 31, 34, 36, 41, 42, 43, 44, 49, 52, 66, 70
Genome Integrity, 43
Genomic Imprinting, 45
genomics, 67
germ cell(s), viii, 4, 8, 13, 14, 15, 23, 27, 32, 33, 34, 36, 38, 39, 40, 41, 43, 44, 46, 49, 50, 51, 52, 53, 54, 56, 57, 59, 60, 61, 62, 63, 66, 68, 69, 71, 72, 73, 74, 75, 76, 77, 78, 79, 81, 82, 83, 84, 87, 88, 90, 93, 97, 99

germ line, 43, 46, 62, 67
glucose, 4, 23
glycosylation, 8
granules, 2, 4, 7, 9, 13, 14, 24, 33, 46, 56
growth, 75, 76, 89, 98
growth arrest, 76
growth factor, 75, 89
GTPases, 6
guanine, 23, 45

H

H3K9me3, 44
hairpin RNAs (hpRNAs), 39, 69
haploid, vii, 2, 32, 33, 44, 49
HBV, 100
heat shock factor 2 (*Hsf2*), 2, 38
heat shock protein, 4, 17
Hen1-mediated 2′-O-methylation, 41
heterochromatin protein 1α (Hp1a), 44
heterogeneity, 93
histology, 15, 27
histone(s), 30, 32, 33, 44, 48
histone 3 lysine 9 (H3K9me3), 44
HIV, 86, 100
homeostasis, viii, 38, 72, 86, 87, 92
HongrES2, 48, 50
hormone(s), 29, 89
HPV, 100
human genome, 35, 47, 58, 66

I

IFN, 83, 85
IFN-β, 83
immune defense, 72, 87
immune function, viii, 71
immune response, viii, 71, 73, 74, 75, 77, 80, 85, 88
immune system, 72, 89, 98
immunity, 74, 91
immunization, 77
immunosuppression, 89
imprinting, 34, 45
in vitro, 14, 51, 81, 90, 93, 95, 96, 99
in vivo, 22, 94, 97
inducible protein, 83, 97, 98
induction, 33, 74, 75, 76, 77, 78, 79, 86, 92
infection, 85, 86, 99
infertility, viii, 2, 16, 20, 38, 39, 52, 62, 72, 73, 78, 80, 86, 87, 88, 92, 94, 100
inflammation, 75, 78, 79, 81, 87, 89, 93, 94, 96, 97
inflammatory responses, 76, 77, 79, 82
infliximab, 97
influenza a, 86
inhibition, 29, 80
inhibitor, 8, 30, 95, 96, 97
initiation, 8, 38, 45
innate immune response(s), 72, 76, 77, 83, 84, 85, 91, 92, 98, 99
innate immunity, 86, 87, 88, 97
integration, 52
integrin, 96
integrity, 34, 43, 44, 70
interface, 10, 13, 18, 20
interferon, 83, 97, 98, 99
intermitochondrial cement (IMC), 33, 46
intracisternal A-particle (IAP), 40, 43
intron(s), 47
IP-10, 98

K

keratin, 10, 12, 26
kidney, 24, 73

L

labeling, 14
large intergenic ncRNAs, 47, 67
lariat introns (ciRNAs), 47
leptotene, 33
leucine, 46
leukemia, 38, 46
leukocytes, 77, 78, 88, 93
ligand, 75, 82, 85, 90, 91, 97, 98
linear lncRNAs, 47

liver, 17, 24
lncRNAdb, 48, 65
localization, 10, 21, 47, 63
loci, 35, 44
locus, 38, 45, 68
long interspersed nuclear elements (LINEs), 40
long noncoding RNAs (lncRNAs), vii, viii, 31, 32, 34, 35, 44, 46, 47, 48, 49, 50, 51, 57, 61, 65, 67, 68, 69, 70
long terminal repeats (LTRs), 40
lumen, 38
lung cancer, 30
Luo, 23, 36, 62, 63
luteinizing hormone, 96
lymph node, 73, 79, 94
lymphocytes, 77, 78, 79, 81, 93, 96
lysine, 44, 48
lysine (K)-specific demethylase 1A (Lsd1), 48

M

m6A modification, 36
machinery, 7, 8, 14, 19, 41, 45, 47, 58, 72, 83
macrophages, 75, 77, 79, 80, 81, 87, 90, 92, 93, 95, 96
male fertility, vii, 1, 18, 24, 35, 39, 65, 68, 70, 72, 73, 85, 86, 87, 92
mammalian cells, 35
mammals, 15, 36, 39, 56, 58, 83
marmoset, 40, 41, 60
mass spectrometry, 14
mast cells, 77, 79
matrix, 20, 26, 97
MCP-1, 82, 98
meiosis, vii, viii, 2, 18, 31, 32, 34, 38, 45, 49, 50, 63, 67, 69, 81
meiosis I, 32
meiosis II, 32
Meiotic Recombination Hot Spot Locus (Mrhl), 50
melanoma, 83
membranes, 5, 6, 7, 8, 10, 25
messenger ribonucleic acid (messenger RNA) (mRNA), 34, 37, 38, 45, 46, 48, 52, 58, 62, 64, 66, 69, 89, 90
metabolism, 4, 36, 37
methyl CpG binding protein 2 (Mecp2), 48
methylated mRNAs, 36, 37
methylation, 33, 35, 37, 41, 43, 44, 45, 48, 52, 53, 54, 55, 59, 61, 65, 68, 69
methyltransferases set domain bifurcated 1 (Setdb1), 44
microorganisms, 72, 84
microprocessor complex, 39
microRNAs (miRNAs), vii, viii, 31, 32, 34, 35, 36, 37, 38, 39, 42, 46, 48, 53, 54, 55, 56, 57, 58, 63, 65, 66, 67, 68, 69
Mili, 33, 40, 41, 42, 43, 45, 46, 56, 68
Ministry of Education, 52
MIP, 82, 97
miRBase, 34, 35
miRNA precursor (pre-miRNAs), 35
miRNA-induced silencing complex (RISC), 36
miRNAs biogenesis, 36
mitochondria, 46, 59, 90
mitogen, 81
mitosis, meiosis, viii, 31, 69
Miwi, 33, 40, 41, 42, 44, 45, 46, 55, 65, 68
Miwi proteins, 41, 42
Miwi/piRNA machinery, 41
Miwi2, 33, 40, 41, 43
mixing, 21
models, 2, 3, 12, 14, 42, 48, 73, 76, 77, 78, 86, 87
modifications, 33, 48
molecular biology, 21
molecules, 44, 48, 59, 74, 94
Moloney leukemia virus 10-like 1 (Mov10l1), 46
monocyte chemoattractant protein (MCP), 82, 97, 98
morphogenesis, vii, 1, 12, 26
morphology, 2, 12, 13
mRNA 5'cap-binding complex, 45
mRNA cleavage, 37, 38, 69
mucin, 8

mucus, 21
mumps, 100
mutagenesis, 43
mutant, 23, 24, 25, 55
mutation(s), 9, 10, 12, 40, 43, 60
myosin, 24

N

narcolepsy, 62
Narcolepsy Candidate-Region 1 Gene (NLC1-C), 49, 51, 62
National Academy of Sciences, 20
National Institutes of Health, 28
natural antisense transcripts (NATs), 47
natural compound, 30
necrosis, 93, 97
neurogenesis, 64
neutrophils, 77
next generation, 43, 47
noncoding RNAs (ncRNAs), vii, viii, 31, 32, 34, 42, 46, 51, 54, 57, 60, 63, 68, 69
nuclear condensation, 32
nuclear membrane, 10, 11, 12, 27
nuclear surface, 2, 4, 5, 7, 10
nucleosomes, 32
nucleotides, 35, 37
nucleus, vii, 1, 2, 7, 10, 11, 12, 21, 26, 27, 35, 37, 43, 44, 50, 51, 63

O

of transition proteins (Tp), 38
omega-3, 21
oocyte, 2, 11
oogenesis, 50
orchitis, viii, 72, 73, 76, 77, 78, 79, 80, 82, 86, 87, 88, 89, 90, 92, 93, 94, 98, 99, 100
organelle(s), 2, 4, 7, 9, 13, 15, 28, 59
ovulation, 96

P

p53, 38, 62
pachytene, 4, 20, 33, 38, 41, 42, 44, 46, 49, 50, 51, 55, 70, 81
pachytene piRNA clusters, 42
pachytene piRNAs, 33, 41, 42, 44, 46, 55
pachytene spermatocytes, 20, 38, 42, 46, 49, 50, 81
pairing, 36, 37, 42, 62
parasites, 72
parathyroid, 73
pathogenesis, 77, 82, 93, 98
pathogens, 72, 82, 84
pathology, 87
pathophysiological, 79, 80
pathway(s), 4, 6, 8, 13, 18, 21, 33, 39, 41, 42, 43, 44, 45, 46, 50, 53, 54, 56, 57, 58, 60, 62, 67, 68, 70, 81, 83, 85, 95, 96, 99
pattern recognition receptors (PRRs), 72, 83
peptidase, 8
permeability, 74, 89
phenotype(s), 4, 5, 11, 38, 43, 78, 79, 90
phosphate, 18, 22, 55
phosphorylation, 12
physical structure, 74
Ping-Pong cycle' pathway, 42
piRNA pathway, 42, 43, 46, 53, 57, 58, 68
piRNA-induced silencing complexes (piRISCs), 42, 43, 44, 45
PIWI Machinery, 40
PIWI proteins, 40, 68
PIWI-interacting RNAs (piRNAs), vii, viii, 31, 32, 33, 34, 39, 40, 41, 42, 43, 44, 45, 46, 52, 57, 58, 60, 62, 64, 68
PIWIL1/HIWI, 40
PIWIL2/HILI, 40
PIWIL3, 40
PIWIL4/HIWI2, 40
plasma membrane, 4, 5, 6, 8, 13, 59
point mutation, 20
polycomb repressive complex 2 (Prc2), 48
polymerase, 35, 62
polypeptide, 46
polyunsaturated fatty acids, 7
population, 45, 78, 93, 94, 98
pre-miRNAs, 35, 37
prepachytene piRNA clusters, 42

prepachytene piRNAs, 41, 42, 43, 44
primary miRNAs (pri-miRNAs), 35, 37
primary piRNAs, 42, 43
primary processing pathway, 42
primary spermatocytes, 17, 32, 51
pro-inflammatory, 78, 80, 81, 82, 83, 84, 86, 87, 97
proliferation, 32, 33, 34, 51, 60, 62, 78, 79, 81, 92, 94
proliferation phase, 32
promoter, 35, 45, 83
promyelocytic leukemia zinc finger gene (*PLZF*), 38, 66
prostatitis, 88
protamines (Prm), 33, 38
proteasome, 41
protein family, 27, 40, 45
protein folding, 4
protein kinases, 26, 81
protein synthesis, 4
proteinase, 79, 94
protein-coding gene(s), 35, 36, 41, 42, 49, 50, 52
proteins, 4, 5, 6, 7, 8, 9, 14, 15, 18, 19, 22, 23, 26, 27, 32, 33, 35, 38, 40, 41, 42, 43, 45, 49, 51, 52, 57, 59, 65, 68, 70, 76, 83, 84, 85, 99
puberty, 72

Q

quality control, 17

R

Rab, 20
Ras protein-specific guanine nucleotide-releasing factor 1 (*Rasgrf1*), 1, 45, 68
receptor(s), 6, 9, 25, 29, 55, 72, 74, 75, 76, 77, 79, 81, 82, 83, 84, 89, 90, 91, 92, 93, 94, 96, 98, 99
recombination, 33
recovery, 29
recycling, 7, 24
regulatory system(s), 77
rejection, 17, 74, 75, 90
remodelling, 19, 60
replication, 84, 85
repression, 34, 37, 43, 62, 64, 67
reproduction, 16, 17, 18, 20, 21, 22, 24, 25, 26, 27, 28, 38
reproductive organs, 95
requirement(s), 70, 100
residues, 82
resolution, 55
retardation, 9
reticulum, 4, 13, 18, 20
retinoblastoma, 54
retinoic acid (RA), 38, 50, 60, 67, 83, 99
retrotransposons, 40, 44
rheumatoid arthritis, 89
ribonucleoprotein (RNP), 45, 47
rings, 13
RISC, 36, 37, 63, 66
RNA, 34, 35, 36, 37, 40, 41, 42, 45, 46, 47, 48, 49, 50, 51, 52, 53, 54, 55, 56, 57, 58, 59, 60, 61, 62, 63, 64, 65, 67, 68, 70, 83
RNA editing, 35, 54
RNA methylation, 35, 52, 55
RNA methyltransferase-like 3 (METTL3), 35
RNA splicing, 47
RNAs, v, viii, 31, 34, 36, 37, 39, 40, 43, 44, 46, 47, 53, 54, 55, 56, 57, 58, 60, 61, 63, 64, 65, 66, 67, 68, 69, 70
RNase III, 35, 62, 69
RNA-seq technology, 41
round spermatids, 6, 12, 32, 33, 38, 40, 42, 46, 49, 50, 51, 81

S

SAM and basic leucine zipper domain containing 1, 46
sclerosis, 79
scrotal, 73
secondary piRNAs, 42, 43
secondary spermatocytes, 32
secretion, 75, 78, 79, 95, 96

self-renewal, vii, 2, 32, 38, 64, 67
seminiferous epithelium, 15, 32, 64, 74, 90, 95, 96
seminiferous tubules, 14, 32, 38, 85
sensing, 98
sensor(s), 10, 83, 85
sequencing, 47, 56, 67
Sertoli cells, 13, 74, 75, 76, 80, 81, 84, 89, 90, 91, 92, 94, 95, 96, 98
shock, 38, 54
signaling pathway, 77, 83
signal/signalling, 15, 25
Silence of Transposons, 43
single-stranded RNA precursors, 42
siRNA, 34, 39, 40, 58
small ncRNAs (sncRNAs), 39, 40, 46, 51
small nucleolar lncRNAs (sno-lncRNAs), 47
small nucleolar RNAs (snoRNAs), 39, 47, 52, 57
somatic cell(s), 9, 40, 81, 82, 89
species, 44, 46, 47, 51
sperm, vii, 1, 2, 12, 13, 15, 16, 18, 22, 25, 26, 27, 33, 44, 50, 51, 59, 64, 87, 91
sperm function, 15, 51
spermatid, 2, 4, 13, 15, 24, 25, 26, 27, 40, 44, 59
spermatids, vii, 2, 6, 7, 8, 9, 11, 12, 13, 15, 17, 19, 20, 24, 26, 32, 33, 38, 40, 44, 46, 85
spermatocyte, 4, 39, 51
spermatogenesis, vii, viii, 1, 2, 14, 15, 16, 17, 18, 20, 21, 23, 24, 26, 29, 30, 31, 32, 33, 34, 35, 36, 38, 39, 40, 41, 43, 45, 46, 49, 50, 51, 54, 55, 56, 57, 58, 59, 61, 62, 63, 64, 65, 66, 67, 68, 69, 70, 71, 72, 74, 76, 79, 80, 81, 82, 87, 88, 89, 91, 92, 94, 97
spermatogenesis and oogenesis-specific basic helix-loop-helix 1 (*Sohlh1*), 50
spermatogonia, viii, 15, 17, 31, 32, 33, 38, 40, 45, 46, 50, 51, 56, 59, 69, 74, 80, 84, 99
spermatogonial stem cells (SSCs), vii, 2, 32, 34, 37, 39, 40, 51, 60, 64, 67
Spermatogonial-Specific lncRNAs (spga-lncRNAs), 51
spermatozoa, vii, viii, 2, 4, 6, 8, 12, 15, 16, 21, 23, 27, 31, 32, 38, 39, 48, 59
spermiogenesis, vii, 2, 6, 7, 12, 15, 17, 18, 19, 20, 22, 23, 24, 26, 27, 32, 33, 34, 38, 46, 51, 54, 58, 65, 68, 69
Sry (sex-determining region Y), 47, 55
SSC fate, 38
stability, 34, 48, 62
sterile, 43, 82
sterols, 18
stimulation, 78, 79, 85, 100
structural changes, 12
structure, 11, 12, 17, 19, 21, 57, 66, 95
Su(var)3–9, 44
suppression, 63, 97
survival, 74, 75, 79, 81, 97
susceptibility, 21, 77
syndrome, 2, 17, 35, 61
synthesis, vii, viii, 4, 7, 18, 32, 72, 79, 80, 81, 82, 84, 85, 95, 96, 97
systemic immune response, 73

T

T cell(s), 75, 78, 79, 87, 89, 93, 98, 100
T lymphocytes, 78
target, 7, 36, 37, 38, 42, 43, 44, 45, 48, 57, 66, 68, 72, 96
target identification, 57
technology, 41, 47
testicular immune privilege, 73
testis, viii, 4, 21, 22, 26, 27, 31, 32, 33, 34, 37, 38, 44, 49, 52, 54, 55, 58, 61, 63, 64, 65, 66, 67, 68, 69, 71, 72, 73, 74, 75, 76, 77, 78, 79, 80, 81, 82, 85, 86, 87, 88, 89, 91, 92, 93, 94, 95, 96, 97, 98, 99
Testis-Specific X-Linked (Tsx), 50, 53
testosterone, 74, 80, 81, 85, 89
therapeutic approaches, 73, 77, 87
therapeutic targets, 15
tissue, viii, 14, 18, 23, 24, 36, 44, 52, 71, 73, 82, 93, 97, 99
TLR, 77, 83, 84, 98

TLR2, 77
TLR3, 83, 84
TLR4, 77, 83, 84
TNF-α, 78, 80, 81, 85, 87, 97
Tp, 38
trafficking, vii, 1, 5, 6, 8, 9, 14, 18, 19, 22, 24, 25
transcription, 15, 33, 34, 35, 38, 43, 47, 48, 50, 54, 56, 57, 59, 60
transcription factors, 15, 48, 59
transcriptome, viii, 31, 34, 52, 60, 63, 66
transferrin, 81, 96
transformation(s), viii, 31, 51
transforming growth factor (TGF), 75, 89, 93
transgene, 53
transition proteins, 32, 33
translation, 34, 38, 45, 48, 55, 67
translation of E2F transcription factor 1 (*E2f1*), 38
transplantation, 93
transport, 4, 5, 6, 8, 9, 12, 14, 18, 19, 23, 24, 25
transport processes, 6
transportation, 5, 7, 9, 10
transposable elements (TEs), 33, 41, 42, 43, 44, 54
treatment, 9, 25, 86, 100
triggers, 51, 85, 95
tropism, 86
tudor domain-containing protein (Tdrd), 45
tumor, 17, 68, 90, 93, 95, 96, 97
tumor necrosis factor (TNF), 78, 80, 81, 85, 87, 90, 93, 95, 96, 97
tyrosine, 12, 26, 27, 50, 76, 91, 92

U

ubiquitin, 8, 23, 29, 41
ubiquitin-26S proteasome (Ub/26S), 41
underlying mechanisms, vii, viii, 72
uridylation, 35

V

vertebrates, 73, 88
vesicle, vii, 1, 5, 6, 7, 9, 14, 18, 19, 21, 22, 24, 25
viral infection, 84, 85, 86, 100
virus infection, 100
viruses, 47, 72, 73, 85, 86
vitamin K, 76

W

Wnt signaling, 50, 53
Wnt signaling pathway, 50

Y

yeast, 28, 47

Z

zinc, 38
zygote, 2